BLACKWELL'S
UNDERGROUND CLINICAL VIGNETTES

MICROBIOLOGY
VOL. II, 3E

BLACKWELL'S
UNDERGROUND CLINICAL VIGNETTES

MICROBIOLOGY
VOL. II, 3E

VIKAS BHUSHAN, MD
University of California, San Francisco, Class of 1991
Series Editor, Diagnostic Radiologist

VISHAL PALL, MBBS
Government Medical College, Chandigarh, India, Class of 1996
Series Editor, U. of Texas, Galveston, Resident in Internal Medicine &
Preventive Medicine

TAO LE, MD
University of California, San Francisco, Class of 1996

HOANG NGUYEN, MD, MBA
Northwestern University, Class of 2001

SONAL SHAH, MD
Ross University, Class of 2000

b

Blackwell
Science

CONTRIBUTORS

Sandra Mun
University of Texas Medical Branch, Class of 2002

Shalin Patel, MD
McGraw Medical Center, Northwestern University, Resident in Internal Medicine

Ashraf Zaman, MBBS
New Delhi, India

Vipal Soni, MD
UCLA School of Medicine, Class of 1999

FACULTY REVIEWER

Warren Levinson, MD, PHD
Professor of Microbiology and Immunology, UCSF School of Medicine

Editorial Offices:

Commerce Place, 350 Main Street, Malden,
    Massachusetts 02148, USA
Osney Mead, Oxford OX2 0EL, England
25 John Street, London WC1N 2BS, England
23 Ainslie Place, Edinburgh EH3 6AJ, Scotland
54 University Street, Carlton, Victoria 3053,
    Australia

Other Editorial Offices:

Blackwell Wissenschafts-Verlag GmbH,
    Kurfürstendamm 57, 10707 Berlin, Germany
Blackwell Science KK, MG Kodenmacho Building,
    7-10 Kodenmacho Nihombashi, Chuo-ku,
    Tokyo 104, Japan
Iowa State University Press, A Blackwell Science
    Company, 2121 S. State Avenue, Ames, Iowa
    50014-8300, USA

Acquisitions: Laura DeYoung
Development: Amy Nuttbrock
Production: Lorna Hind and Shawn Girsberger
Manufacturing: Lisa Flanagan
Marketing Manager: Kathleen Mulcahy
Cover design by Leslie Haimes
Interior design by Shawn Girsberger
Typeset by TechBooks
Printed and bound by Capital City Press

Blackwell's Underground Clinical Vignettes:
    Microbiology II, 3e
ISBN 0-632-04549-3

Printed in the United States of America
02 03 04 05 5 4 3 2 1

First Indian Reprint 2002

Printed and bound by Multivista Global Limited,
Chennai - 600 042.

The Blackwell Science logo is a trade mark of
Blackwell Science Ltd., registered at the United
Kingdom Trade Marks Registry

Library of Congress Cataloging-in-Publication Data
Bhushan, Vikas.
Blackwell's underground clinical vignettes.
Microbiology / Author, Vikas Bhushan.– 3rd ed.
    p. ; cm. – (Underground clinical vignettes)
Rev. ed. of: Microbiology/Vikas Bhushan ... [et al.].
2nd ed. c1999-. ISBN 0-632-04547-7 (alk. paper)
1. Medical microbiology – Case studies.
2. Physicians – Licenses – United States –
Examinations – Study guides.
    [DNLM: 1. Microbiology – Case Report.
2. Microbiology – Problems and Exercises. QW 18.2
B575b 2002] I. Title: Microbiology. II. Title:
Underground clinical vignettes. Microbiology.
III. Microbiology. IV. Title. V. Series.
    QR46 .B465 2002
    616'.01'076–dc21

                                    2001004932

Notice

The authors of this volume have taken care that the information contained herein is accurate and compatible with the standards generally accepted at the time of publication. Nevertheless, it is difficult to ensure that all the information given is entirely accurate for all circumstances. The publisher and authors do not guarantee the contents of this book and disclaim any liability, loss, or damage incurred as a consequence, directly or indirectly, of the use and application of any of the contents of this volume.

CONTENTS

ACKNOWLEDGMENTS

Throughout the production of this book, we have had the support of many friends and colleagues. Special thanks to our support team including Anu Gupta, Andrea Fellows, Anastasia Anderson, Srishti Gupta, Mona Pall, Jonathan Kirsch and Chirag Amin. For prior contributions we thank Gianni Le Nguyen, Tarun Mathur, Alex Grimm, Sonia Santos and Elizabeth Sanders.

We have enjoyed working with a world-class international publishing group at Blackwell Science, including Laura DeYoung, Amy Nuttbrock, Lisa Flanagan, Shawn Girsberger, Lorna Hind and Gordon Tibbitts. For help with securing images for the entire series we also thank Lee Martin, Kristopher Jones, Tina Panizzi and Peter Anderson at the University of Alabama, the Armed Forces Institute of Pathology, and many of our fellow Blackwell Science authors.

For submitting comments, corrections, editing, proofreading, and assistance across all of the vignette titles in all editions, we collectively thank:

Tara Adamovich, Carolyn Alexander, Kris Alden, Henry E. Aryan, Lynman Bacolor, Natalie Barteneva, Dean Bartholomew, Debashish Behera, Sumit Bhatia, Sanjay Bindra, Dave Brinton, Julianne Brown, Alexander Brownie, Tamara Callahan, David Canes, Bryan Casey, Aaron Caughey, Hebert Chen, Jonathan Cheng, Arnold Cheung, Arnold Chin, Simion Chiosea, Yoon Cho, Samuel Chung, Gretchen Conant, Vladimir Coric, Christopher Cosgrove, Ronald Cowan, Karekin R. Cunningham, A. Sean Dalley, Rama Dandamudi, Sunit Das, Ryan Armando Dave, John David, Emmanuel de la Cruz, Robert DeMello, Navneet Dhillon, Sharmila Dissanaike, David Donson, Adolf Etchegaray, Alea Eusebio, Priscilla A. Frase, David Frenz, Kristin Gaumer, Yohannes Gebreegziabher, Anil Gehi, Tony George, L.M. Gotanco, Parul Goyal, Alex Grimm, Rajeev Gupta, Ahmad Halim, Sue Hall, David Hasselbacher, Tamra Heimert, Michelle Higley, Dan Hoit, Eric Jackson, Tim Jackson, Sundar Jayaraman, Pei-Ni Jone, Aarchan Joshi, Rajni K. Jutla, Faiyaz Kapadi, Seth Karp, Aaron S. Kesselheim, Sana Khan, Andrew Pin-wei Ko, Francis Kong, Paul Konitzky, Warren S. Krackov, Benjamin H.S. Lau, Ann LaCasce, Connie Lee, Scott Lee, Guillermo Lehmann, Kevin Leung, Paul Levett, Warren Levinson, Eric Ley, Ken Lin,

Pavel Lobanov, J. Mark Maddox, Aram Mardian, Samir Mehta, Gil Melmed, Joe Messina, Robert Mosca, Michael Murphy, Vivek Nandkarni, Siva Naraynan, Carvell Nguyen, Linh Nguyen, Deanna Nobleza, Craig Nodurft, George Noumi, Darin T. Okuda, Adam L. Palance, Paul Pamphrus, Jinha Park, Sonny Patel, Ricardo Pietrobon, Riva L. Rahl, Aashita Randeria, Rachan Reddy, Beatriu Reig, Marilou Reyes, Jeremy Richmon, Tai Roe, Rick Roller, Rajiv Roy, Diego Ruiz, Anthony Russell, Sanjay Sahgal, Urmimala Sarkar, John Schilling, Isabell Schmitt, Daren Schuhmacher, Sonal Shah, Fadi Abu Shahin, Mae Sheikh-Ali, Edie Shen, Justin Smith, John Stulak, Lillian Su, Julie Sundaram, Rita Suri, Seth Sweetser, Antonio Talayero, Merita Tan, Mark Tanaka, Eric Taylor, Jess Thompson, Indi Trehan, Raymond Turner, Okafo Uchenna, Eric Uyguanco, Richa Varma, John Wages, Alan Wang, Eunice Wang, Andy Weiss, Amy Williams, Brian Yang, Hany Zaky, Ashraf Zaman and David Zipf.

For generously contributing images to the entire *Underground Clinical Vignette* Step 1 series, we collectively thank the staff at Blackwell Science in Oxford, Boston, and Berlin as well as:

- Axford, J. *Medicine.* Osney Mead: Blackwell Science Ltd, 1996. Figures 2.14, 2.15, 2.16, 2.27, 2.28, 2.31, 2.35, 2.36, 2.38, 2.43, 2.65a, 2.65b, 2.65c, 2.103b, 2.105b, 3.20b, 3.21, 8.27, 8.27b, 8.77b, 8.77c, 10.81b, 10.96a, 12.28a, 14.6, 14.16, 14.50.

- Bannister B, Begg N, Gillespie S. *Infectious Disease, 2ⁿᵈ Edition.* Osney Mead: Blackwell Science Ltd, 2000. Figures 2.8, 3.4, 5.28, 18.10, W5.32, W5.6.

- Berg D. *Advanced Clinical Skills and Physical Diagnosis.* Blackwell Science Ltd., 1999. Figures 7.10, 7.12, 7.13, 7.2, 7.3, 7.7, 7.8, 7.9, 8.1, 8.2, 8.4, 8.5, 9.2, 10.2, 11.3, 11.5, 12.6.

- Cuschieri A, Hennessy TPJ, Greenhalgh RM, Rowley DA, Grace PA. *Clinical Surgery.* Osney Mead: Blackwell Science Ltd, 1996. Figures 13.19, 18.22, 18.33.

- Gillespie SH, Bamford K. *Medical Microbiology and Infection at a Glance.* Osney Mead: Blackwell Science Ltd, 2000. Figures 20, 23.

- Ginsberg L. *Lecture Notes on Neurology, 7ᵗʰ Edition.* Osney Mead: Blackwell Science Ltd, 1999. Figures 12.3, 18.3, 18.3b.

- Elliott T, Hastings M, Desselberger U. *Lecture Notes on Medical Microbiology, 3ʳᵈ Edition.* Osney Mead: Blackwell Science Ltd, 1997. Figures 2, 5, 7, 8, 9, 11, 12, 14, 15, 16, 17, 19, 20, 25, 26, 27, 29, 30, 34, 35, 52.

- Mehta AB, Hoffbrand AV. *Haematology at a Glance*. Osney Mead: Blackwell Science Ltd, 2000. Figures 22.1, 22.2, 22.3.

Please let us know if your name has been missed or misspelled and we will be happy to make the update in the next edition.

PREFACE TO THE 3RD EDITION

We were very pleased with the overwhelmingly positive student feedback for the 2nd edition of our *Underground Clinical Vignettes* series. Well over 100,000 copies of the UCV books are in print and have been used by students all over the world.

Over the last two years we have accumulated and incorporated **over a thousand "updates"** and improvements suggested by you, our readers, including:

- many additions of specific boards and wards testable content

- deletions of redundant and overlapping cases

- reordering and reorganization of all cases in both series

- a new master index by case name in each Atlas

- correction of a few factual errors

- diagnosis and treatment updates

- addition of 5–20 new cases in every book

- and the addition of clinical exam photographs within *UCV— Anatomy*

And most important of all, the third edition sets now include two brand new **COLOR ATLAS** supplements, one for each Clinical Vignette series.

- The *UCV–Basic Science Color Atlas* (*Step 1*) includes over 250 color plates, divided into gross pathology, microscopic pathology (histology), hematology, and microbiology (smears).

- The *UCV–Clinical Science Color Atlas* (*Step 2*) has over 125 color plates, including patient images, dermatology, and funduscopy.

Each atlas image is descriptively captioned and linked to its corresponding Step 1 case, Step 2 case, and/or Step 2 MiniCase.

How Atlas Links Work:

Step 1 Book Codes are:
A = Anatomy
BS = Behavioral Science
BC = Biochemistry
M1 = Microbiology, Vol. I
M2 = Microbiology, Vol. II
P1 = Pathophysiology, Vol. I
P2 = Pathophysiology, Vol. II
P3 = Pathophysiology, Vol. III
PH = Pharmacology

Step 2 Book Codes are:
ER = Emergency Medicine
IM1 = Internal Medicine, Vol. I
IM2 = Internal Medicine, Vol. II
NEU = Neurology
OB = OB/GYN
PED = Pediatrics
SUR = Surgery
PSY = Psychiatry
MC = MiniCase

Case Number

UCV1 M-P3-032A   UCV2 ER-035A, ER-035B

Indicates Type of Image:
H = Hematology
M = Microbiology
PG = Gross Pathology
PM = Microscopic Pathology

Indicates UCV1 or UCV2 Series

- If the Case number (032, 035, etc.) is not followed by a letter, then there is only one image. Otherwise A, B, C, D indicate up to 4 images.

Bold Faced Links: In order to give you access to the largest number of images possible, we have chosen to cross link the Step 1 and 2 series.

- If the link is bold-faced this indicates that the link is direct (i.e., Step 1 Case with the Basic Science Step 1 Atlas link).

- If the link is not bold-faced this indicates that the link is indirect (Step 1 case with Clinical Science Step 2 Atlas link or vice versa).

We have also implemented a few structural changes upon your request:

- Each current and future edition of our popular *First Aid for the USMLE Step 1* (Appleton & Lange/McGraw-Hill) and *First Aid for the USMLE Step 2* (Appleton & Lange/McGraw-Hill) book will be linked to the corresponding UCV case.

- We eliminated UCV → First Aid links as they frequently become out of date, as the *First Aid* books are revised yearly.

- The Color Atlas is also specially designed for quizzing—captions are descriptive and do not give away the case name directly.

We hope the updated UCV series will remain a unique and well-integrated study tool that provides compact clinical correlations to basic science information. They are designed to be easy and fun (comparatively) to read, and helpful for both licensing exams and the wards.

We invite your corrections and suggestions for the fourth edition of these books. For the first submission of each factual correction or new vignette that is selected for inclusion in the fourth edition, you will receive a personal acknowledgment in the revised book. If you submit over 20 high-quality corrections, additions or new vignettes we will also consider **inviting you to become a "Contributor" on the book of your choice**. If you are interested in becoming a potential "Contributor" or "Author" on a future UCV book, or working with our team in developing additional books, please also e-mail us your CV/resume.

We prefer that you submit corrections or suggestions via electronic mail to **UCVteam@yahoo.com**. Please include "Underground Vignettes" as the subject of your message. If you do not have access to e-mail, use the following mailing address: Blackwell Publishing, Attn: UCV Editors, 350 Main Street, Malden, MA 02148, USA.

Vikas Bhushan
Vishal Pall
Tao Le
October 2001

HOW TO USE THIS BOOK

This series was originally developed to address the increasing number of clinical vignette questions on medical examinations, including the USMLE Step 1 and Step 2. It is also designed to supplement and complement the popular *First Aid for the USMLE Step 1* (Appleton & Lange/McGraw Hill) and *First Aid for the USMLE Step 2* (Appleton & Lange/McGraw Hill).

Each UCV 1 book uses a series of approximately 100 **"supra-prototypical" cases as a way to condense testable facts and associations**. The clinical vignettes in this series are designed to incorporate as many testable facts as possible into a cohesive and memorable clinical picture. The vignettes represent composites drawn from general and specialty textbooks, reference books, thousands of USMLE style questions and the personal experience of the authors and reviewers.

Although each case tends to present all the signs, symptoms, and diagnostic findings for a particular illness, **patients generally will not present with such a "complete" picture either clinically or on a medical examination**. Cases are not meant to simulate a potential real patient or an exam vignette. All the **boldfaced "buzzwords" are for learning purposes** and are not necessarily expected to be found in any one patient with the disease.

Definitions of selected important terms are placed within the vignettes in (SMALL CAPS) in parentheses. Other parenthetical remarks often refer to the pathophysiology or mechanism of disease. The format should also help students learn to present cases succinctly during oral "bullet" presentations on clinical rotations. The cases are meant to serve as a condensed review, not as a primary reference. The information provided in this book has been prepared with a great deal of thought and careful research. This book should not, however, be considered as your sole source of information. Corrections, suggestions and submissions of new cases are encouraged and will be acknowledged and incorporated when appropriate in future editions.

ABBREVIATIONS

5-ASA	5-aminosalicylic acid
ABGs	arterial blood gases
ABVD	adriamycin/bleomycin/vincristine/dacarbazine
ACE	angiotensin-converting enzyme
ACTH	adrenocorticotropic hormone
ADH	antidiuretic hormone
AFP	alpha fetal protein
AI	aortic insufficiency
AIDS	acquired immunodeficiency syndrome
ALL	acute lymphocytic leukemia
ALT	alanine transaminase
AML	acute myelogenous leukemia
ANA	antinuclear antibody
ARDS	adult respiratory distress syndrome
ASD	atrial septal defect
ASO	anti-streptolysin O
AST	aspartate transaminase
AV	arteriovenous
BE	barium enema
BP	blood pressure
BUN	blood urea notrogen
CAD	coronary artery disease
CALLA	common acute lymphoblastic leukemia antigen
CBC	complete blood count
CHF	congestive heart failure
CK	creatine kinase
CLL	chronic lymphocytic leukemia
CML	chronic myelogenous leukemia
CMV	cytomegalovirus
CNS	central nervous system
COPD	chronic obstructive pulmonary disease
CPK	creatine phosphokinase
CSF	cerebrospinal fluid
CT	computed tomography
CVA	cerebrovascular accident
CXR	chest x-ray
DIC	disseminated intravascular coagulation
DIP	distal interphalangeal
DKA	diabetic ketoacidosis
DM	diabetes mellitus
DTRs	deep tendon reflexes
DVT	deep venous thrombosis

EBV	Epstein–Barr virus
ECG	electrocardiography
Echo	echocardiography
EF	ejection fraction
EGD	esophagogastroduodenoscopy
EMG	electromyography
ERCP	endoscopic retrograde cholangiopancreatography
ESR	erythrocyte sedimentation rate
FEV	forced expiratory volume
FNA	fine needle aspiration
FTA-ABS	fluorescent treponemal antibody absorption
FVC	forced vital capacity
GFR	glomerular filtration rate
GH	growth hormone
GI	gastrointestinal
GM-CSF	granulocyte macrophage colony stimulating factor
GU	genitourinary
HAV	hepatitis A virus
hcG	human chorionic gonadotrophin
HEENT	head, eyes, ears, nose, and throat
HIV	human immunodeficiency virus
HLA	human leukocyte antigen
HPI	history of present illness
HR	heart rate
HRIG	human rabies immune globulin
HS	hereditary spherocytosis
ID/CC	identification and chief complaint
IDDM	insulin-dependent diabetes mellitus
Ig	immunoglobulin
IGF	insulin-like growth factor
IM	intramuscular
JVP	jugular venous pressure
KUB	kidneys/ureter/bladder
LDH	lactate dehydrogenase
LES	lower esophageal sphincter
LFTs	liver function tests
LP	lumbar puncture
LV	left ventricular
LVH	left ventricular hypertrophy
Lytes	electrolytes
MCHC	mean corpuscular hemoglobin concentration
MCV	mean corpuscular volume
MEN	multiple endocrine neoplasia

MGUS	monoclonal gammopathy of undetermined significance
MHC	major histocompatibility complex
MI	myocardial infarction
MOPP	mechlorethamine/vincristine (Onçovorin)/ procarbazine/prednisone
MR	magnetic resonance (imaging)
NHL	non-Hodgkin's lymphoma
NIDDM	non-insulin-dependent diabetes mellitus
NPO	nil per os (nothing by mouth)
NSAID	nonsteroidal anti-inflammatory drug
PA	posteroanterior
PIP	proximal interphalangeal
PBS	peripheral blood smear
PE	physical exam
PFTs	pulmonary function tests
PMI	point of maximal intensity
PMN	polymorphonuclear leukocyte
PT	prothrombin time
PTCA	percutaneous transluminal angioplasty
PTH	parathyroid hormone
PTT	partial thromboplastin time
PUD	peptic ulcer disease
RBC	red blood cell
RPR	rapid plasma reagin
RR	respiratory rate
RS	Reed–Sternberg (cell)
RV	right ventricular
RVH	right ventricular hypertrophy
SBFT	small bowel follow-through
SIADH	syndrome of inappropriate secretion of ADH
SLE	systemic lupus erythematosus
STD	sexually transmitted disease
TFTs	thyroid function tests
tPA	tissue plasminogen activator
TSH	thyroid-stimulating hormone
TIBC	total iron-binding capacity
TIPS	transjugular intrahepatic portosystemic shunt
TPO	thyroid peroxidase
TSH	thyroid-stimulating hormone
TTP	thrombotic thrombocytopenic purpura
UA	urinalysis
UGI	upper GI
US	ultrasound

VDRL   Venereal Disease Research Laboratory
VS   vital signs
VT   ventricular tachycardia
WBC   white blood cell
WPW   Wolff–Parkinson–White (syndrome)
XR   x-ray

ID/CC A 30-year-old female presents to the ER with **severe**, sudden-onset **shortness of breath** and an **extensive** pruritic **skin rash**.

HPI She was **prescribed cotrimoxazole** by her general physician for a UTI; she took the **first dose only a few minutes before** developing symptoms.

PE VS: **hypotension**. PE: severe **respiratory distress**; central cyanosis; extensive **urticarial wheals** noted all over body.

Labs **IgE antibody** demonstrated to sulfonamides by **RAST**.

Treatment **Epinephrine** (1:1000); antihistaminics; steroids; ventilatory support; adequate IV fluid administration or vasopressor agents to treat hypotension.

Discussion Systemic anaphylaxis is the most serious and life-threatening **IgE-mediated type I hypersensitivity reaction**; its recognition and prompt treatment are critical to survival.

ID/CC A **2-year-old male** is admitted to the hospital for evaluation of a suspected immune disorder.

HPI He has a history of **recurrent fungal** diaper rashes and **staphylococcal cervical furunculosis** requiring multiple incisions and drainage in addition to antibiotics. His mother also reports chronic diarrhea and a prior perianal fistula.

PE Cervical lymphadenopathy; mild hepatomegaly and splenomegaly; no pallor, purpuric patches, or sternal tenderness.

Labs CBC/PBS: **neutrophilic leukocytosis**. Elevated ESR; normal serum immunoglobulins; **absence of respiratory burst** (negative nitroblue tetrazolium test and chemoluminescence assay); negative Mantoux test.

Imaging CXR: hilar lymphadenopathy. US, abdomen: hepatosplenomegaly; hepatic and splenic nodular lesions (due to granulomas).

Micro Pathology Characteristic granuloma formation with phagocytes, giant cells, and occasional histiocytes in lymph nodes, liver, spleen, and lungs.

Treatment Long-term TMP-SMX prophylaxis, γ-interferon.

Discussion Chronic granulomatous disease is most commonly an **X-linked** disorder of neutrophil function (may have variable inheritance patterns) that is due to a **deficiency of NADPH oxidase**. Neutrophils of affected patients demonstrate normal chemotaxis, degranulation, and phagocytosis but cannot use the oxygen-dependent myeloperoxidase system for microbial killing, making patients susceptible to recurrent staphylococcal infections.

ID/CC	A 19-year-old male has **recurrent attacks** of bilateral **periorbital and hand swelling** coupled with **respiratory difficulty that lasts up to 24 hours** and often requires hospitalization.
HPI	He does not, however, complain of itching. His **father** and his **aunt** both suffer from a **similar illness**.
PE	Physical examination unremarkable.
Labs	**Decreased C4** (best screening test); **decreased C1 inhibitor** (confirmatory test) and C2; normal C3; normal IgE.
Treatment	Synthetic androgens (e.g., danazol), fresh frozen plasma.
Discussion	C1 esterase inhibitor deficiency is inherited as an **autosomal-dominant** trait; **death** may result from **laryngeal edema**. Also known as hereditary angioedema.

HEREDITARY ANGIOEDEMA

ID/CC	A 25-year-old **white** female is referred to an internist by her family doctor for a workup of **recurrent sinusitis**, chronic otitis media, one episode of **pneumonia** that required hospitalization, and recurrent bouts of watery **diarrhea**.
HPI	She has seen an allergy specialist for several years and has received desensitization shots for **multiple allergies**, including pollen, dust, and cat hair.
PE	Normal except for **hypopigmented spots on neck and arms** (VITILIGO).
Labs	**Markedly decreased serum IgA; normal IgG and IgM.**
Imaging	XR, sinus: opacification of paranasal sinuses (due to chronic sinusitis).
Treatment	Largely supportive; antibiotic therapy; try to **avoid blood or plasma transfusion** (anaphylaxis or serum sickness due to presence of antibodies to IgA).
Discussion	Selected IgA deficiency is the **most common congenital immunodeficiency**, especially in patients of European descent. Diarrhea is usually caused by *Giardia lamblia*; recurrent sinopulmonary infections are caused by *Streptococcus pneumoniae, Haemophilus influenzae*, or *Staphylococcus aureus*; associated with an increased incidence of allergies and autoimmune diseases such as SLE and rheumatoid arthritis. Selective IgA deficiency may be due to a specific defect in isotype switching.

SELECTIVE IgA DEFICIENCY

ID/CC	A **4-month-old male** presents with **chronic diarrhea** and **failure to thrive**.
HPI	The infant was diagnosed with extensive **mucocutaneous candidiasis** in the early neonatal period and shortly thereafter developed a fulminant *Pseudomonas* **septicemia** that required intravenous antibiotic therapy for an extended period of time. A paternal cousin had developed similar and equally devastating bacterial and fungal infections in the neonatal period and subsequently died.
PE	Emaciated; mucocutaneous **candidiasis** noted; **tonsils not seen; lymph nodes not palpable** despite recurrent infections.
Labs	CBC: severe lymphopenia. PBS: **lack of mature lymphocytes**. Tests for cutaneous **delayed hypersensitivity** and contact sensitization negative; **serum immunoglobulin levels** (IgG, IgA, and IgM) **low; adenosine deaminase (ADA) deficiency** demonstrated in red cells.
Imaging	CXR: **absent thymic shadow**.
Gross Pathology	Thymus fails to descend into the anterior mediastinum from the neck and resembles fetal thymus of 6 to 8 weeks.
Micro Pathology	No lymphoid tissue in the lymph nodes, spleen, tonsils, and appendix.
Treatment	**Bone marrow transplant** from an HLA-identical sibling; IV immunoglobulin; infusion of normal ADA-containing erythrocytes (ADA-PEG is also very successful); antibiotics; gene therapy for ADA; genetic counseling (SCID caused by ADA deficiency can be diagnosed prenatally by amniocentesis).
Discussion	Severe combined immunodeficiency syndrome is characterized by marked depletion of the cells that mediate both humoral (B-cell) and cellular (T-cell) immunity. SCID may be transmitted as either an autosomal-recessive trait or an X-linked recessive trait, or it may be sporadic; half of the cases inherited in an **autosomal-recessive** manner are caused by a **deficiency in ADA**.

SEVERE COMBINED IMMUNODEFICIENCY (SCID)

ID/CC	A 7-month-old **male** is admitted for a workup of **recurrent upper respiratory tract and skin infections** of several months' duration.
HPI	His parents state that he has had recurrent URIs, one episode of *Haemophilus influenzae* **pneumonia**, and severe otitis media.
PE	Low weight and height for chronological age; chronic bilateral suppurative otitis media; **asymmetric arthritis** of knees; **no tonsillar tissue** seen; no lymphadenopathy or hepatosplenomegaly.
Labs	**Panhypogammaglobulinemia: very low** IgG; IgA and IgM undetectable.
Treatment	Parenteral gamma globulin; monitor pulmonary function to guard against chronic lung disease.
Discussion	An X-linked disease (manifests **only in males**) characterized by a **selective B-cell defect** with **recurrent bacterial infections**. Also known as **Bruton's disease**, X-linked hypogammaglobulinemia is due to a genetic defect in tyrosine kinase receptor found on antibody precursors, resulting in impaired maturation and development of antibodies. Male infants demonstrate infections when maternal antibodies have cleared from their system.

ID/CC A 27-year-old white female complains of **mouth ulcers, prolonged fever**, flulike symptoms, and increasing fatigue and weight loss over the past 2 months.

HPI She recently moved from a large metropolitan area to a farm in **Ohio**, where she spent 1 week cleaning a **pigeons' loft**.

PE VS: fever (38.5°C). PE: pallor; weight loss; enlarged liver and spleen; generalized lymphadenopathy; scattered sibilant rales over lung fields.

Labs CBC/PBS: anemia; leukopenia. Small, budding fungus found **intracellularly in reticuloendothelial cells** (macrophages) on silver stain; elevated LDH; positive blood culture for dimorphic fungus.

Imaging CXR: nonsegmental shifting pneumonic infiltrates; mediastinal adenopathy with popcorn calcifications; bilateral **hilar adenopathy**. CT, abdomen: splenic calcifications.

Gross Pathology Nodules with granuloma formation; central area of necrosis and caseation with sclerosis and calcification; any organ may be involved, mainly reticuloendothelial system (RES) and adrenals.

Micro Pathology **Granulomas** with epithelioid cells, Langhans' giant cells, and organisms within macrophages; in disseminated disease, organisms present in RES throughout body with proliferation.

Treatment Itraconazole; amphotericin B.

Discussion Histoplasmosis is a systemic fungal infection sometimes resembling TB that is caused by *Histoplasma capsulatum*, a dimorphic fungus. The yeast form is found intracellularly; the mold form is found in soil associated with **bird or bat feces**. Transmitted by inhalation of mold spores, it varies in intensity from asymptomatic to fulminant (in immunocompromised patients). The disease is most prevalent in the southeastern, mid-Atlantic, and central regions of the United States.

ID/CC	A 57-year-old **black** male complains to his doctor of increasing weakness, **swollen glands in the armpits and groin**, and a feeling of **heaviness in the abdomen** (due to hepatosplenomegaly).
HPI	The patient is an immigrant from **Trinidad and Tobago** and has a history of nonresolving skin rashes and recurrent respiratory infections.
PE	Marked **pallor**; extensive papular skin rash with few erythematous plaques over abdomen; **generalized lymphadenopathy and hepatosplenomegaly**.
Labs	CBC/PBS: marked **leukocytosis** (83,000) with relative **lymphocytosis** and **atypical lymphocytes. Increased LDH; hypercalcemia**.
Imaging	CXR: normal.
Micro Pathology	Skin biopsy reveals infiltration by **leukemic CD4+ T lymphocytes**.
Treatment	Aggressive combination chemotherapy.
Discussion	Adult T-cell leukemia/lymphoma (ATLL) is associated with HTLV-1 type C, a retrovirus that has a higher incidence in **blacks** from the **Caribbean and southeastern United States** as well as in people from **southern Japan and sub-Saharan Africa**. The infection is acquired via transmission from mother to child (breast milk), from sexual activity, from blood transfusion, or from IV drug use.

ID/CC A **2-day-old** neonate is evaluated for an **eye discharge**.

HPI The baby's **mother is a prostitute** who did not receive any prenatal cervical cultures during pregnancy.

PE Normal full-term male neonate; mucoid **eye discharge, conjunctival congestion, and chemosis** noted in both eyes; nonfollicles seen on palpebral conjunctiva (due to absence of subconjunctival adenoid layer at this age); mild **superficial keratitis** also present.

Labs Gram stain of swab reveals increased **PMNs** and **no bacteria**; characteristic **intracellular inclusion bodies demonstrated by the DIF test**; cell culture yields *Chlamydia trachomatis* serotypes D through K; chlamydia also grown from **maternal cervical swab**.

Treatment **Erythromycin syrup; azithromycin suspension** has also been shown to be beneficial; no topical therapy.

Discussion *Chlamydia trachomatis* is an important cause of preventable blindness; its strains can be further differentiated into 18 serotypes by microimmunofluorescence tests. **Serotypes A, B, Ba, and C** are principally associated with **endemic trachoma** in developing countries; **serotypes D through K** primarily cause **sexually transmitted** infections in adults and **inclusion conjunctivitis and pneumonia in infants**, transmitted through an infected birth canal; and **serotypes L1, L2, and L3** cause **lymphogranuloma venereum**.

INCLUSION CONJUNCTIVITIS

ID/CC A 20-year-old male college student complains of **sore throat, fatigue, fever, swollen lymph nodes on the back of his neck**, anorexia, cough, and **malaise** of 10 days' duration.

HPI He was initially given **ampicillin** by his school nurse, after which he developed an extensive **skin rash**.

PE VS: fever. PE: enlargement of submaxillary and **cervical lymph nodes; exudative tonsillitis**; petechiae on soft palate; slightly **enlarged spleen and liver**.

Labs CBC/PBS: anemia; thrombocytopenia; leukocytosis with absolute **lymphocytosis** (50%); **atypical lymphocytes**. Elevated ALT, AST, and bilirubin; **positive heterophil antibody test** (PAUL-BUNNELL TEST); IgM antibodies to viral capsid antigen/monospot positive.

Gross Pathology Enlarged spleen, lymph nodes, and, to lesser extent, liver; hepatitis may be present along with brain involvement; splenic rupture rare complication.

Micro Pathology Proliferation of reticuloendothelial system; infiltration of spleen by atypical lymphocytes.

Treatment **Supportive**.

Discussion Infectious mononucleosis is a systemic viral infection that is caused by Epstein–Barr virus (EBV), a herpesvirus, and is transmitted through respiratory droplets and saliva. In developed countries, it most commonly affects teenagers and young adults ("kissing disease"); in underdeveloped countries, it is seen as a subclinical infection of early childhood. EBV infection is associated with an increased risk of **Burkitt's lymphoma, Hodgkin's disease**, and **nasopharyngeal carcinoma**.

Atlas Links UCV1 H-M2-010   UCV2 IM2-022

ID/CC	A 65-year-old male presents with a **high fever**, headache, extreme prostration, a **nonproductive cough**, and severe **breathlessness**.
HPI	He had been receiving chlorambucil for treatment of chronic lymphocytic leukemia (CLL) and was in an extremely **debilitated state**.
PE	VS: fever; tachypnea; cyanosis. PE: **conjunctival congestion; pharyngeal inflammation; rales and wheezes** heard on auscultation over both lung fields; splenomegaly and lymphadenopathy (due to CLL).
Labs	No organisms seen or cultured from sputum; fluorescent antibody directed against **influenza virus** was positive; viral cultures of nasopharyngeal washings grew influenza virus; fourfold rise in **hemagglutination inhibition antibody titer** against influenza virus demonstrated.
Imaging	CXR (PA view): bilateral, diffuse interstitial infiltrates suggestive of **atypical pneumonia**.
Treatment	**Amantidine or rimantadine** for influenza A (**zanamivir or oseltamivir** for influenza A and B); ventilatory support, antipyretics, and IV fluids. **Secondary staphylococcal pneumonia** should be treated with parenteral antibiotics; **yearly vaccination** prevents excessive morbidity and mortality, especially among the elderly.
Discussion	Influenza viruses are medium-sized spherical **RNA viruses termed orthomyxoviruses**; influenza A and B viruses each contain 8 RNA segments and 10 viral proteins. Influenza infection is **most common in winter**, with the **severity** of a given **outbreak depending on the status of immunity** in the community. Previous natural infection or immunization with viruses that are immunologically close to the current strain limits new infection, but if **antigenic drift** results in reduced cross-reactivity, the new strain will spread more rapidly. New strains produced by **antigenic shift** account for most major outbreaks. Influenza affects all segments of the population, but severe infections and **major complications** are most common **in patients who are young, elderly, or debilitated**.

ID/CC	A 30-year-old female presents with **fever, chills**, malaise, headaches, and **myalgias**.
HPI	She was diagnosed as suffering from **secondary syphilis** with an extensive nonpruritic **skin rash, condylomata lata**, and **mucous patches** in the mouth, for which she received a dose of intramuscular **penicillin 6 hours ago**.
PE	VS: **fever**; tachycardia; mild hypotension.
Treatment	**No specific treatment**; symptoms subside in 24 hours.
Discussion	The Jarisch-Herxheimer reaction consists of fever, chills, mild hypotension, headache, and an increase in the intensity of mucocutaneous lesions **2 hours after** initiating **treatment of syphilis with penicillin** or another effective antibiotic; symptoms usually **subside in 12 to 24 hours**. The reaction occurs in 50% of patients with primary syphilis and in 90% of those with secondary syphilis. The Jarisch-Herxheimer reaction **also occurs after treatment of other spirochetal diseases** (e.g., louse-borne relapsing fever caused by *Borrelia recurrentis*). It has been suggested that the release of treponemal lipopolysaccharides might produce this symptom complex.

ID/CC A 40-year-old male smoker complains of acute-onset **high fever**, chills, a **nonproductive cough**, tachypnea, and **pleuritic chest pain**.

HPI A number of **similar cases** have been reported in his workplace in recent months. The patient admits to significant alcohol and tobacco consumption and uses a **humidifier** at night.

PE VS: fever; dyspnea. PE: rales present bilaterally on auscultation.

Labs Sputum exam with Gram stain reveals no pathogenic organisms. CBC: neutrophilic leukocytosis. Cold agglutinins absent; indirect fluorescent antibody technique reveals stable titer of > 1:256 (considered diagnostic); **direct immunofluorescent** staining of sputum confirms presence of *Legionella*.

Imaging CXR, PA: bilateral diffuse, patchy infiltrates and **ill-defined nodules**.

Gross Pathology Nodular areas of consolidation that may progress to involvement of one or more lobes of the lung.

Micro Pathology Alveolar exudate with PMNs, macrophages, and fibrin; in more severe cases, destruction of alveolar septa.

Treatment Erythromycin or an active fluoroquinolone.

Discussion Legionnaire's disease is caused by *Legionella pneumophila*, a filamentous, flagellated, aerobic gram-negative, motile bacillus, and is more common in immunocompromised patients. Epidemiologic studies have established **drinking water** and **air conditioners** as the sources of outbreak.

ID/CC A 30-year-old **Pakistani immigrant** complains of chronic **fever**, weight loss, increased abdominal girth, a feeling of heaviness, and appetite loss.

HPI Almost a year ago, the patient had a small, pruritic red **papule** on his left arm that was caused by an insect bite and disappeared spontaneously.

PE **Skin darkening**; trophic changes in hair; **massive** nontender, hard **splenomegaly**; hepatomegaly without jaundice; generalized lymphadenopathy; peripheral edema; ecchymosis.

Labs CBC/PBS: **anemia, leukopenia, thrombocytopenia** (PANCYTOPENIA), and monocytosis; **amastigotes in buffy coat**. Hypergammaglobulinemia; decreased albumin; increased ALT and AST.

Imaging CT/US, abdomen: splenomegaly.

Gross Pathology **Massively enlarged spleen**; also greatly increased in weight, dark colored, and congested with Leishman–Donovan bodies.

Micro Pathology Proliferation of reticuloendothelial system cells; biopsy or aspiration reveals parasite-filled macrophages in infected locations.

Treatment Pentavalent antimony (e.g., **sodium stibogluconate**); amphotericin B or pentamidine isethionate.

Discussion Also known as kala azar, leishmaniasis is a zoonosis that is produced by *Leishmania donovani* and is transmitted through the bite of the *Phlebotomus* **sandfly**. It is associated with a high fatality rate when left untreated.

Atlas Links ⬜UCV1 M-M2-014A, M-M2-014B, M-M2-014C, H-M2-014

ID/CC A 30-year-old male from **India** presents with slowly progressive **hypopigmented skin patches and nodules** together with a peculiar **deformity of the nose.**

HPI The patient has a history of **nasal stuffiness** and bloody nasal discharge; he also complains of **loss of libido.**

PE **Leonine facies** (thickened facial and forehead skin); loss of eyebrows and eyelashes (MADAROSIS); scleral nodules; **depressed nasal bridge** ("SADDLE-NOSE" DEFORMITY); gynecomastia; **testicular atrophy**; numerous **symmetrical, hypopigmented macules with vague edges** and erythematous, smooth, shiny surfaces; skin plaques and nodules; **partial loss of pinprick and temperature sensation** (HYPOESTHESIA); no anhidrotic changes; symmetrically **enlarged ulnar and common peroneal nerves.**

Labs CBC: mild anemia. ESR elevated; slit skin smears reveal **numerous acid-fast bacilli** on modified ZN staining.

Micro Pathology Dermis massively and diffusely infiltrated with **foamy histiocytes with bacilli and globi** (masses of acid-fast bacilli) containing Virchow giant cells; bacilli found only rarely in epidermis and in subepidermal **"clear zone"**; epidermis thinned out with flattening of rete ridges.

Treatment Multidrug therapy with **rifampicin, dapsone, and clofazimine.**

Discussion The discovery of one or more of the following is pathognomonic of leprosy: (1) **anesthetic skin lesions** (found in all tuberculoid and many lepromatous cases); (2) **thickening of one or more nerves** (found in many lepromatous and some tuberculoid cases); and (3) the presence of **acid-fast bacilli in skin smears** (found in all lepromatous and some tuberculoid cases). *Mycobacterium leprae* has not been cultured in vitro thus far. Frequent complications include hand crippling (secondary to nerve damage) and blindness. It is currently believed that in most instances, the mode of transmission is via person-to-person contact.

Atlas Links UCV2 MC-179A, MC-179B

ID/CC	A 26-year-old male from India presents with a **hypopigmented, anesthetic skin patch** over the left side of his face.
HPI	He also complains of an occasional "electric current"-like sensation radiating from his left elbow to his hand.
PE	Dry, hypopigmented, anesthetic patch over left cheek; left **ulnar nerve enlarged and palpable**; eye, ear, nose, and throat exam normal; testes normal (vs. signs that are often demonstrable in lepromatous leprosy).
Labs	Glucose-6-phosphate dehydrogenase (G6PD) levels within normal range (done to prevent dapsone-associated hemolysis); slit skin smears reveal few **acid-fast bacilli**; skin biopsy from patch diagnostic of tuberculoid leprosy.
Gross Pathology	**Single or small number of lesions** with macular or raised edges.
Micro Pathology	Skin biopsy reveals many well-formed epithelioid granulomas with very **few** acid-fast bacilli.
Treatment	Chemotherapy with rifampin and dapsone.
Discussion	Caused by *Mycobacterium leprae*, an acid-fast bacillus. The organism has two unique properties: it is thermolabile, growing best at 27°C to 30°C, and it divides very slowly; generation time is 12 to 14 days. Consequently, leprosy in humans typically evolves very slowly. Tuberculoid leprosy predominantly affects the skin with limited nerve involvement (most commonly ulnar and peroneal); **lepromatous leprosy** has diffuse involvement of the skin, eyes, nerves, and upper airway with disfigurement of the hands and face (**leonine facies**).
Atlas Links	UCV2 MC-179A, MC-179B

ID/CC A 35-year-old British **dairy farmer** complains of a high remittent **fever** with chills, severe muscle aches, **decreased urine output**, and **dark-colored urine** for the past 2 days.

HPI He also complains of an extensive skin rash and nasal bleeding (EPISTAXIS). A careful history reveals that the area in which he works is infested with rodents.

PE VS: **fever**; tachycardia; hypotension. PE: **icterus**; extensive hemorrhagic maculopapular skin eruption; **conjunctival suffusion**; lymphadenopathy.

Labs CBC: leukocytosis with neutrophilia; thrombocytopenia. Mild **hyperbilirubinemia**, predominantly conjugated; **increased alkaline phosphatase; elevated BUN and creatinine**. UA: proteinuria, **casts**, and RBCs. Blood culture (positive during first 10 days of illness) and urine culture (positive after second week of infection) on Fletcher's medium isolated *Leptospira interrogans*; serologic diagnosis (positive during second week of illness): microscopic slide agglutination demonstrated significant titer of antibody to *L. interrogans*.

Imaging CXR: patchy alveolar infiltrates consistent with alveolar hemorrhage.

Gross Pathology Severe infection damages both the **liver and kidneys**.

Micro Pathology Liver biopsy shows focal centrilobular necrosis with focal lymphocytic infiltration and disorganization of liver cell plates together with proliferation of Kupffer cells with cholestasis; kidney biopsy reveals mesangial proliferation with PMN infiltration.

Treatment Penicillin (dose modified due to presence of renal failure), doxycycline; hemodialysis.

Discussion Weil's disease, a severe form of leptospirosis caused by *Leptospira interrogans* complex, is characterized by fever, jaundice, cutaneous and visceral hemorrhages, anemia, azotemia, and altered consciousness; major vectors to humans are rodents. Transmission occurs through direct contact with the blood, tissue, or urine of infected animals. Person-to-person transmission is highly unlikely. Preventive measures include limiting the rodent population and vaccinating animals.

17 LEPTOSPIROSIS (WEIL'S DISEASE)

ID/CC	A **2-week-old** female is brought to the emergency room because of **high fever and convulsions**.
HPI	She also has an **extensive skin rash** on her legs and trunk.
PE	VS: fever. PE: generalized hypotonia; **extensive maculopapular skin rash; nuchal rigidity; involuntary flexion of hips when flexing neck** (BRUDZINSKI'S SIGN).
Labs	CBC: neutrophilic leukocytosis. LP: elevated CSF cell count (750 cells/mL), mostly **neutrophils**; elevated CSF protein; low CSF sugar. Gram-positive, facultative, intracellular, nonsporulating motile bacilli on Gram stain and culture.
Gross Pathology	Purulent meningitis.
Micro Pathology	Bacillus provokes both acute suppurative reaction with neutrophilic infiltration and chronic granuloma formation with focal necrosis.
Treatment	IV antibiotics (high-dose ampicillin).
Discussion	Listeriosis is caused by *Listeria monocytogenes*. Bacterial infection may occur early (acquired **in utero**) or later (drinking **contaminated milk**) in neonatal life. May be rapidly fatal if disseminated. Also occurs in adults immunocompromised by disease (e.g., renal disease or HIV). *Escherichia coli* and group B streptococcus are two other common causes of neonatal meningitis.

ID/CC	A 12-year-old male presents with **fatigue, fever**, headache, **fleeting joint pain**, and a **reddish rash** on his trunk and left leg of 1 week's duration.
HPI	The patient is a native of **Connecticut** and attended a summer camp in the state's national park 2 weeks ago. He recalls having noticed a **tick bite** on his leg about 2 weeks ago.
PE	VS: fever. PE: red macule on site of bite that has grown circumferentially; **active border and central clearing** (ERYTHEMA CHRONICUM MIGRANS); femoral lymphadenopathy; mild neck stiffness; normal CNS exam.
Labs	**Positive IgM ELISA** for *Borrelia burgdorferi*; diagnosis confirmed by Western blot assay. ECG: normal. LP: lymphocytic pleocytosis; increased proteins. *B. burgdorferi* grown on Noguchi medium.
Gross Pathology	Erythema chronicum migrans (ECM) is characteristic of Lyme disease; must be minimum of 5 cm in diameter for diagnosis to be made; center may desquamate, ulcerate, or necrose; satellite lesions sometimes seen; may spontaneously disappear with time.
Treatment	**Doxycycline**; amoxicillin; ceftriaxone.
Discussion	The most common disease transmitted by vectors in the United States, Lyme disease is caused by *Borrelia burgdorferi*, a spirochete, and is transmitted through *Ixodes* species tick bites. Ticks acquire *B. burgdorferi* from deer mice, which are the natural reservoir. There are three recognized stages: stage 1 consists of ECM and constitutional symptoms; stage 2, cardiac or neurologic involvement; and stage 3, persistent migratory arthritis, synovitis, and **atrophic patches on the distal extremities** (ACRODERMATITIS CHRONICUM ATROPHICANS).

ID/CC	A 57-year-old black female from Kenya complains of increasing weight and **edema of the lower legs** with difficulty walking.
HPI	Over the years she has had episodes of **fever with swelling of inguinal lymph nodes** and itching. She has also had numerous attacks of malaria.
PE	Inguinal lymph nodes indurated and slightly increased in size; marked deformity in both legs with **thickening of skin** and greatly **increased diameter; rubbery consistency**.
Labs	PBS: several **microfilariae**; prominent **eosinophilia**.
Imaging	Lymphangiogram: partial lymphatic obstruction at iliac level.
Gross Pathology	Presence of adult worms in lymphatics; marked fibrosis surrounding obstructed vessels.
Micro Pathology	Granulomatous reaction with plasma cell and lymphocytic infiltration; giant cell formation; intense fibroblastic hyperplasia.
Treatment	**Ivermectin; diethylcarbamazine**; surgery in advanced cases.
Discussion	Lymphatic filariasis is a chronic disease that is due to lymphatic obstruction and is caused by several types of filarial roundworms, mainly *Wuchereria bancrofti* and *Brugia malayi*; it is transmitted by female **mosquito bites**. Also known as elephantiasis.
Atlas Link	ⓊⒸⓋⓘ M-M2-020

ID/CC . A 25-year-old male complains of swollen, **tender masses in his groin** and very painful **genital ulcers** of 1 week's duration.

HPI The patient admits to having had **unprotected sex** with multiple partners.

PE **Swollen**, erythematous, tender **inguinal nodes**, usually bilateral, with draining sinuses (INGUINAL ADENITIS, BUBOES); multiple small genital lesions.

Labs Inguinal node biopsy diagnostic; **positive complement fixation test; positive immunofluorescence test**.

Gross Pathology Primary lesion is ulcerated nodule; gives rise to **inguinal bubo**, an enlarged lymph node sometimes characterized by fistulous tract formation; balanitis, phimosis, and rectal involvement with stricture may also be present.

Micro Pathology Neutrophilic infiltration of primary lesion with areas of necrosis; lymphoid hyperplasia of lymph nodes with foci of macrophage accumulation; abscess formation with fibrosis.

Treatment **Doxycycline**; tetracycline; azithromycin; erythromycin; TMP-SMX; ceftriaxone; ciprofloxacin.

Discussion Lymphogranuloma venereum is an STD that is due to *Chlamydia trachomatis* (**L1, L2, L3**). Counseling should be given about other STDs (e.g., AIDS, syphilis, gonorrhea).

ID/CC	A 30-year-old missionary comes to the emergency room complaining of **high fever, chills, severe headache**, and confusion.
HPI	Upon returning from **Africa** 2 weeks ago, he began to feel weak and experienced backaches, pain behind the eyes, and sleepiness.
PE	VS: fever (39°C); tachycardia. PE: pallor; profuse **sweating**; mild splenomegaly without lymphadenopathy.
Labs	CBC/PBS: anemia; thrombocytopenia; **plasmodia in erythrocytes on thick peripheral blood smear**. Slight hyperbilirubinemia and hypoglycemia.
Gross Pathology	Liver and spleen moderately enlarged and soft in consistency, with sequestration and hemolysis of erythrocytes and macrophages; hyperplasia of Kupffer cells; malarial pigment in spleen and liver; brain capillaries may show thromboses.
Micro Pathology	Hypertrophy of phagocytic system; ischemic necrosis surrounding occluded blood vessels in brain.
Treatment	Chloroquine; quinine for cerebral malaria; sulfadiazine-pyrimethamine, mefloquine, tetracycline for areas with chloroquine-resistant strains; primaquine for radical treatment.
Discussion	Malaria is transmitted by female *Anopheles* **mosquitoes**. *Plasmodium falciparum* may be lethal, producing cerebral malaria. Other types include *P. vivax, P. ovale,* and *P. malariae*.
Atlas Links	[U][C][V] H-M2-022A, H-M2-022B, H-M2-022C

ID/CC	A **3-year-old** female is brought to the emergency room with a **high fever of 7 days' duration**, accompanied by **redness of the eyes**, persistent dry **cough**, and **coryza**.
HPI	Her family doctor had treated her illness as a viral URI, but no improvement was seen. One day before her admission, her mother noticed a **skin rash starting behind her ears and face** that has now spread to her trunk and extremities.
PE	Pallor; injected conjunctiva; hyperemic throat; erythematous maculopapular rash on face, neck, trunk, and extremities; retroauricular lymphadenopathy; **bluish-gray spots surrounded by erythematous areola on buccal mucosa in region of first molar** (KOPLIK'S SPOTS).
Labs	CBC: **leukopenia**.
Gross Pathology	**Koplik's spots** pathognomonic of measles; appearance presages rash by approximately 2 days; uniform lesions (vs. varicella).
Micro Pathology	Lymphocytic dermal infiltration; multinucleated giant cells in reticuloendothelial system (WARTHIN-FINKELDEY CELLS).
Treatment	No specific antiviral therapy available; treat complications.
Discussion	Also called **rubeola**; not to be confused with rubella. Measles is produced by a **paramyxovirus** and is transmitted by **respiratory droplets**; a live attenuated vaccine is available. Measles has an incubation period of 10 to 14 days. Sequelae include encephalitis, subacute sclerosing panencephalitis (SSPE), and giant cell pneumonia.
Atlas Links	UCV2 PED-030A, PED-030B

ID/CC A 12-year-old white female is brought to the emergency room because of sudden **fever** with **chills, severe headache**, pain in the extremities and back, **stiff neck**, and generalized rash; she also **fainted** while in school.

HPI She had been well until admission, with no relevant history. In the emergency room, she **vomits bright red blood** twice.

PE VS: tachycardia; hypotension (BP 70/50). PE: altered sensorium; pallor; moist, cold skin; nuchal rigidity and positive Kernig's sign; **petechial rash** all over body; minimal papilledema on funduscopic exam; no focal neurologic signs.

Labs **Hypoglycemia**. Lytes: **hyponatremia; hyperkalemia**. CBC/PBS: thrombocytopenia; **neutrophilic leukocytosis**. LP: **CSF** cloudy and under increased pressure; increased proteins; low sugar. **Gram-negative diplococci** (*Neisseria meningitidis*) **seen within and outside WBCs** on Gram stain; negative India ink and ZN stain; growth of meningococci later revealed on blood culture.

Imaging CT, head: normal. CT, abdomen: bilateral adrenal hemorrhage.

Gross Pathology **Bilateral adrenal hemorrhagic necrosis**; skin necrosis; pyogenic meningitis.

Micro Pathology Meningeal hyperemia with abundant purulent exudate; diplococcus-containing PMNs; acute hemorrhagic necrosis of adrenal glands.

Treatment Steroid replacement; IV fluids; dopamine; IV penicillin G; prophylactic rifampin for close contacts.

Discussion Meningococcemia is a **fulminant disease** caused by several groups of *Neisseria meningitidis*; the cause of death is adrenal necrosis with vascular collapse. A meningococcal vaccine is available. Also known as **Waterhouse–Friderichsen syndrome**.

Atlas Link 🅄🄲🅅2 IM2-024

ID/CC	A 24-year-old white female with **insulin-dependent diabetes mellitus (IDDM)** is hospitalized for **ketoacidosis** following a night out drinking; on the fifth day she develops right **periorbital swelling** and a mucopurulent postnasal discharge that **fails to respond to antibiotics**.
HPI	She admits to irregular adherence to glucose control and insulin dosing.
PE	Right **periorbital** and paranasal **edema**; swelling of conjunctiva (CHEMOSIS); exophthalmos; **black ulceration of nasal mucosa; third cranial nerve** (CN III) **palsy**.
Labs	**Large, irregular, nonseptate hyphae branching at wide (> 90°) angles** on nasal culture.
Imaging	XR, plain: opacification of paranasal sinuses.
Gross Pathology	Necrotic destruction of paranasal sinuses and orbit with dissemination to lung and brain.
Micro Pathology	Purulent arteritis with thrombi composed of hyphae; inflammation and necrosis with polymorphonuclear infiltrate.
Treatment	Maintain tighter glucose control; **amphotericin B**; surgical drainage.
Discussion	Mucormycosis is a phycomycosis produced by *Mucor* and *Rhizopus* molds; it should be suspected in cases of antibiotic-resistant sinusitis, especially in the presence of underlying diabetes, burns, lymphoma, or leukemia.
Atlas Link	UCV1 M-M2-025

MUCORMYCOSIS

ID/CC	A **6-year-old** white male presents with fever, nausea, vomiting, **swelling**, and tenderness of the **mandibular angle**; he finds it difficult to talk, eat, or swallow.
HPI	Two of his classmates were diagnosed with mumps 2 weeks ago. There is no vaccination record.
PE	VS: fever. PE: outward and upward displacement of ear; **obliterated mandibular hollow; orifice of Stensen's duct swollen and hyperemic; right testicle enlarged and painful**.
Labs	CBC: leukopenia with **lymphocytosis. Hyperamylasemia**; positive complement fixation antibodies.
Gross Pathology	Parotid glands enlarged with areas of necrosis and mononuclear infiltrate; encephalitis, orchitis, oophoritis, meningitis, and pancreatitis may also be present.
Micro Pathology	Examination of parotid glands reveals perivascular mononuclear, lymphocytic, and plasma cell infiltrate with necrosis; ductal obstruction and edema; testicular interstitial edema; perivascular cerebral lymphocytic cuffing.
Treatment	Supportive; analgesics for pain; treat complications.
Discussion	A systemic infection caused by the mumps virus, an RNA paramyxovirus, mumps is transmitted by droplets and direct contact. Bilateral testicular involvement may lead to sterility; one of the most common causes of pancreatitis in children. A vaccine is available with measles and rubella (MMR).

ID/CC	A 20-year-old male college student presents with a **productive cough**, headache, **malaise**, runny nose, and **fever**.
HPI	He has a history of sore throat preceding the onset of the **cough, which initially was nonproductive**.
PE	VS: fever. PE: mild respiratory distress; auscultation reveals fine to medium rales over right lower lobe.
Labs	Gram stain of sputum negative; routine cultures of both blood and sputum negative. CBC: **leukocyte count normal**. Fourfold rise in complement fixation titer in paired sera; **cold agglutinin titer > 1:128**.
Imaging	CXR: patchy alveolar infiltrates involving right lower lobe; appears worse than the clinical picture.
Gross Pathology	Unilateral lower lobe pneumonia with firm, red pulmonary parenchyma in affected areas.
Micro Pathology	Bronchial mucosa congested and edematous; inflammatory response consists of perivascular lymphocytes initially and PMNs later in infection. **Organism lacks cell wall** (thus penicillins and cephalosporins are ineffective).
Treatment	**Erythromycin.**
Discussion	*Mycoplasma pneumoniae* is the **most common cause of primary atypical pneumonia**. Transmission is by droplet spread; rapidly infects those living in close quarters.

MYCOPLASMA PNEUMONIA

ID/CC　A 50-year-old diabetic male presents with **fever, pain, and a necrotizing swelling** over his left leg.

HPI　His symptoms began about a week ago with redness and swelling of the left leg followed by bronze discoloration of the skin and the appearance of hemorrhagic bullae.

PE　Extensive cutaneous **gangrene** observed over left leg with many ruptured bullae; black necrotic eschar with surrounding erythema resembles a third-degree burn.

Labs　Swab staining reveals presence of chains of gram-positive cocci; culture isolated **β-hemolytic group A streptococcus** (*Streptococcus pyogenes*).

Micro Pathology　Biopsy specimen reveals areas of necrosis in dermis and subcutaneous fat, infiltration with PMNs, and vasculitis and thrombosis in vessels in the superficial fascia.

Treatment　Treatment includes rapid **surgical excision of necrotic tissue** in combination with appropriate **antibiotics**.

Discussion　Streptococcal gangrene is a group A streptococcal cellulitis that rapidly progresses to gangrene of the subcutaneous tissue and necrosis of the overlying skin; the disease process usually involves an extremity. Necrotizing fasciitis is also recognized as a polymicrobial infection that is caused by aerobes and anaerobes ("SYNERGISTIC NECROTIZING CELLULITIS"). Infection spreads quickly through various fascial planes, the venous system, and lymphatics. Predisposing etiologies include surgery, trauma, and diabetes.

ID/CC A 45-year-old white male undergoing **chemotherapy** for Hodgkin's lymphoma is brought to the emergency room by his wife because of shortness of breath and cyanosis.

HPI For the past **3 months**, he has been complaining of intermittent weakness, fever with chills, and foul-smelling, thick **greenish sputum**.

PE VS: fever (38°C); tachypnea; tachycardia. PE: pallor; mild cyanosis; localized dullness with bronchial breathing; diminished breath sounds over left lower lobe.

Labs CBC: leukocytosis with neutrophilia; anemia. Sputum culture reveals **gram-positive, filamentous, partially acid-fast** staining bacteria (due to *Nocardia*).

Imaging CXR: nodular infiltrate in left lower lobe with air-fluid level (abscess) and left pleural effusion.

Gross Pathology Lung lesions or disseminated lesions (brain, liver, kidney, subcutaneous tissue) consist of necrotic centers within regions of consolidation and abscess formation resembling pyogenic pneumonia.

Micro Pathology Consolidation of alveoli with pus formation (exudate of PMNs and fibrin) and surrounding granulomatous reaction.

Treatment Six-month course of TMP-SMX; surgery.

Discussion A chronic bacterial infection seen in diabetics, leukemia and lymphoma patients, and **immunocompromised patients**, nocardiosis usually involves the lungs with possible dissemination to the brain, subcutaneous tissue, and other organs. It is caused by *Nocardia asteroides*, a branching, aerobic, gram-positive organism that is weakly acid fast and is sometimes confused with *Mycobacterium tuberculosis*.

ID/CC   A 60-year-old male who was hospitalized following a stroke presents with a high-grade **fever with chills** and obtundation.

HPI   He had been **catheterized due to urinary incontinence and was receiving cephalosporin** for treatment of aspiration pneumonitis.

PE   VS: fever.

Labs   **Blood culture** grew *Enterococcus fecalis* (morphologically indistinguishable from streptococci and immunologically similar to members of group D streptococci, the enterococci are metabolically unique in their ability to resist heat, bile, and 6.5% NaCl); urine culture also isolated *Streptococcus fecalis*.

Treatment   **Ampicillin with gentamicin** (**vancomycin** can be substituted for ampicillin in patients with penicillin allergies).

Discussion   Enterococci constitute a relatively common cause of UTIs, wound infections, and peritonitis and intra-abdominal abscesses; they have also become an increasingly prominent cause of **bacteremia**, which usually originates from a **focus in the urinary tract or abdomen**. The incidence of nosocomial bacteremias caused by these organisms is also increasing, particularly in patients who have received cephalosporins or other broad-spectrum antibiotics. All clinically significant isolates should be subjected to testing for β-**lactamase production,** high-level **aminoglycoside resistance**, and **vancomycin resistance** to determine if an alternative therapy is necessary. Infections caused by enterococci that produce β-lactamase are treated with an antimicrobial agent that combines a penicillin with a β-lactamase inhibitor; infections caused by strains that are highly resistant to aminoglycosides are treated with vancomycin.

ID/CC A 56-year-old white female is referred to an ophthalmologist for an evaluation of **diminished visual acuity**.

HPI She has spent most of her adult life as a missionary in rural **Senegal** and **Mali**. She admits to chronic **generalized itching, mostly while showering**.

PE Wrinkling and loss of elastic tissue in skin; **marked hypopigmentation of shins**; 2- to 3-cm, nonfixed, firm, nontender subcutaneous **nodules on iliac bones, knees, and elbows**; chronic conjunctivitis, **sclerosing keratitis, and chorioretinal lesions** on eye exam.

Labs CBC/PBS: **eosinophilia**. Fifty-milligram dose of **diethylcarbamazine produces severe pruritus, rash, fever, and conjunctivitis** (POSITIVE MAZZOTTI REACTION).

Micro Pathology Skin biopsy at iliac crest shows microfilariae.

Treatment **Ivermectin**; suramin.

Discussion Onchocerciasis is caused by *Onchocerca volvulus* and is transmitted by the blackfly (*SIMULIUM*), which breeds near rivers; hence it is also known as **"river blindness."** Larvae migrate through subcutaneous tissue, producing **painless soft tissue edema** (CALABAR EDEMA); with time, subcutaneous nodules form and filariae obstruct dermal lymphatics, producing atrophy and hypopigmentation. Microfilariae concentrate in the eyes, leading to **chorioretinitis and blindness**.

ID/CC   A 9-year-old male is admitted for an evaluation of a **suspected** underlying **immune deficiency**.

HPI   He has been hospitalized and treated several times for **recurrent life-threatening septicemia due to *Streptococcus pneumoniae*, meningococcus**, and *Haemophilus influenzae*. Careful history reveals that a few years ago he underwent an emergency **splenectomy** following traumatic splenic rupture in a motor vehicle accident.

PE   Left paramedian postsurgical scar seen on abdomen.

Labs   Reduced IgM levels; **reduced antibody production when challenged with particulate antigens**; PBS reveals **Howell–Jolly bodies**.

Imaging   US, abdomen: **spleen** is **absent**.

Treatment   **Pneumococcal vaccine and prophylactic antibiotics** (penicillin, amoxicillin, TMP-SMX).

Discussion   Patients who have undergone **splenectomy or** who are **functionally asplenic** are at increased **risk for overwhelming bacteremia**; pathogens include **organisms that possess a polysaccharide capsule**, such as meningococcus, *Staphylococcus*, the DF2 bacillus, and, especially, *Streptococcus pneumoniae* and *Haemophilus influenzae* type B. Such **functionally asplenic** patients include individuals with **sickle cell disease** and those who have undergone **splenic irradiation. Pneumococcal vaccine** is indicated in all patients who have undergone splenectomy, particularly children and adolescents.

ID/CC   A 12-year-old girl arrives in the emergency room with **pain, swelling, and limited motion** of her left hand; she also complains of fever and chills.

HPI   The girl was **bitten by a cat** yesterday while playing at a friend's house.

PE   Hand is erythematous, **shiny**, and **markedly edematous**; on palpation, hand is **tender** with fluctuation (cellulitis); limited passive and active motion; yellowish-green **purulent fluid** drains from wound; left epitrochlear and axillary **lymphadenitis** without lymphangitis.

Labs   **Gram-negative rods with bipolar staining** of abscess aspirate; **catalase and oxidase positive** (*Pasteurella multocida*).

Imaging   XR, plain: soft tissue swelling; no periostitis or erosions (vs. osteomyelitis).

Treatment   **Incision and drainage, amoxicillin/clavulanate**; tetracycline; penicillin.

Discussion   *Pasteurella multocida* is the most common bacterium isolated from cat bite wounds and may progress to **osteomyelitis**. Human bite infections are most commonly caused by *Eikenella corrodens* and are treated with penicillin.

ID/CC	A 44-year-old male archaeologist presents with **high fever, malaise**, intense **headache, severe myalgia**, and **painful swelling in the inguinal region**.
HPI	He recently returned from a trip to **Arizona**.
PE	VS: tachycardia. PE: drowsy looking; no meningeal signs; pustule seen at site of an **insect bite** on left upper arm; **inguinal lymph nodes enlarged, fluctuant, and tender** (BUBOES); no lesion on external genitalia.
Labs	CBC/PBS: normal; no malarial parasites. Gram-negative bacilli with **"safety pin"** appearance seen in aspirates from buboes; culture of aspirate reveals *Yersinia pestis*.
Gross Pathology	Enlarged lymph nodes are necrotic and suppurative; pneumonic form shows lobar consolidation.
Micro Pathology	Numerous organisms in suppurative and necrotic lymph tissue.
Treatment	Streptomycin; gentamicin; doxycycline prophylaxis for close contacts; tetracycline.
Discussion	Plague is usually acquired after contact with **rodents and fleas** in endemic areas (southwestern United States). Septic shock, pneumonia, DIC, and vascular collapse are life-threatening sequelae. Death rapidly ensues in the absence of treatment.

ID/CC	An 11-year-old white male presents with a high-grade fever, a productive, **blood-tinged** cough, **mucoid sputum**, and **pleuritic left-sided chest pain** of a few days' duration.
HPI	The child had previously been well and is fully immunized.
PE	VS: fever; tachypnea. PE: use of accessory respiratory muscles; central trachea; decreased left respiratory excursion; **increased vocal fremitus in left infrascapular area with dullness to percussion; bronchial breathing** with coarse crackles heard over left lung area.
Labs	CBC: increased WBC count; preponderance of neutrophils. ABGs: hypoxemia without hypercapnia. **Gram-positive diplococci in sputum**; α-hemolytic colonies of gram-positive diplococci (*Streptococcus pneumoniae*) on blood agar culture.
Imaging	CXR: **homogenous opacification of left lower lobe** (LOBAR CONSOLIDATION) with small left pleural effusion.
Gross Pathology	Consolidation of lung parenchyma passes through four stages: congestion and edema, red hepatization, gray hepatization, and resolution.
Micro Pathology	Vascular dilatation with hyperemia and alveolar edema; PMNs rich in purulent exudate; fibrin deposition; hardening of lung parenchyma with fibrin clotting inside alveoli (consolidation).
Treatment	Parenteral therapy with penicillin; monitor with radiologic imaging; supplemental oxygen for respiratory distress.
Discussion	*S. pneumoniae* is the most common cause of community-acquired pneumonia and produces typical lobar pneumonia.
Atlas Links	UCV1 M-M2-035A, M-M2-035B, M-M2-035C, PG-M2-035

ID/CC	A 32-year-old **HIV-positive male** presents with **progressively increasing dyspnea** over the past 3 weeks.
HPI	He also complains of a **dry**, painful **cough**, marked **fatigue**, and a continuous **low-grade fever**. He has been noncompliant with cotrimoxazole prophylaxis.
PE	VS: fever; marked **tachypnea**. PE: pallor; generalized lymphadenopathy; respiratory distress; **intercostal retraction**; mild central cyanosis; nasal flaring; coarse, crepitant rales auscultated at both lung bases.
Labs	ABGs: **hypoxemia out of proportion to clinical findings**. *Pneumocystis carinii* on **methenamine silver stain** of induced sputum or bronchoalveolar lavage; ELISA/Western blot positive for HIV. CBC: **leukopenia** with depressed CD4+ cell count. **Serum LDH typically elevated**.
Imaging	CXR: diffuse, bilaterally symmetrical **interstitial and alveolar infiltration** pattern, predominantly perihilar; no lymphadenopathy or effusion.
Gross Pathology	Congestion and consolidation of lungs with hypoaeration.
Micro Pathology	Eosinophilic exudate in alveoli with multiple 4- to 6-mm cysts containing oval bodies (MEROZOITES) on lung biopsy or bronchial lavage; *Pneumocystis* abundant on Gomori methenamine silver stain.
Treatment	**TMP-SMX**; pentamidine; steroids for severe disease.
Discussion	*Pneumocystis carinii* pneumonia is an opportunistic infection that causes interstitial pneumonia in many **immunocompromised** patients. Traditionally it has been classified as a protozoan; however, *P. carinii* ribosomal RNA indicates that the organism is **fungal**. It is seen in the upper lobes in patients receiving inhaled pentamidine prophylaxis. Treat HIV patients prophylactically with TMP-SMX for *P. carinii* pneumonia if the CD4 count is < 200.
Atlas Links	⬜UCV1 M-M2-036A, M-M2-036B, M-M2-036C

ID/CC A 25-year-old HIV-negative **homosexual male** presents with rectal burning, itching in the anal region, **diarrhea, tenesmus**, and a **bloody, mucopurulent discharge** per rectum.

HPI One month ago he was hospitalized with severe **febrile proctocolitis** that was diagnosed as **lymphogranuloma venereum**. He has also been treated several times in the past for amebiasis and shigella colitis and admits to having **receptive anal intercourse**. Further history reveals that his most recent **sexual partner** has been suffering from **urethral pain and discharge**.

PE Condylomata acuminata noted in perianal distribution; remainder of physical exam normal.

Labs Gram stain and culture of **rectal swab** reveals gram-negative diplococci identified as *Neisseria gonorrhoeae* on Thayer-Martin medium; urethral swab from partner also isolates *N. gonorrhoeae*.

Imaging Sigmoidoscopy: proctitis with bloody mucopurulent discharge noted.

Treatment **Ceftriaxone** and **doxycycline** (to treat likely concomitant chlamydial infection) for both patient and partner. Most apparent failures of correct antibiotic therapy are in fact due to reinfection; in resistant cases, **spectinomycin, fluoroquinolones**, or other **cephalosporins** can be used.

Discussion The term **"gay bowel syndrome"** is used in reference to enteric and perirectal infections that are commonly encountered in immune-competent homosexual men; in homosexuals with HIV, opportunistic organisms play a more important role. Common etiologic agents include *Chlamydia trachomatis*, lymphogranuloma venereum serovars, *Neisseria gonorrhoeae*, HSV, *Treponema pallidum*, human papillomavirus, *Campylobacter* species, *Shigella*, *Entamoeba histolytica*, and *Giardia*.

ID/CC	A 35-year-old male presents with high **fever**, malaise, headache, and a **hacking cough productive** of a small amount of mucoid sputum.
HPI	He has two **pet parrots** at home who have recently shown **signs of illness**.
PE	VS: fever; **bradycardia**. PE: auscultation of chest reveals **crepitant rales** over both lower lung fields; **splenomegaly** with mild hepatomegaly noted; multiple **purpuric macules** seen over abdomen ("HORDER'S SPOTS").
Labs	Greater than fourfold rise in complement-fixing antibody titer to a group antigen suggestive of infection with *Chlamydia psittaci*; definitive diagnosis of psittacosis was made from sputum by isolation of *C. psittaci* in pretreated tissue culture cells.
Imaging	CXR, PA: **interstitial** patchy, bilateral **infiltrates**.
Gross Pathology	Principal lesions found in lungs, liver and spleen.
Micro Pathology	Pulmonary lesion is an **interstitial pneumonitis**; mononuclear cells with ballooned cytoplasm containing inclusion bodies are observed. In the liver, focal necrosis of hepatocyte occurs along with Kupffer cell hyperplasia.
Treatment	**Azithromycin** or **clarithromycin**.
Discussion	Psittacosis is an acute infection caused by *Chlamydia psittaci*; it is characterized primarily by pneumonitis and systemic manifestations and is **transmitted** to humans by a variety of avian species, **principally psittacine birds (parrots, parakeets)**. A history of contact with birds, particularly sick birds, or of employment in a pet shop or in the poultry industry provides a clue to the diagnosis of psittacosis in a patient with pneumonia, especially if bradycardia and splenomegaly are also present.

ID/CC   A 54-year-old **female** being treated in the ER is noted to have developed **progressively worsening abdominal pain and high-grade fever with chills**.

HPI   She presented to the ER a few hours ago with colicky abdominal pain and was diagnosed with **choledocholithiasis**.

PE   VS: **fever** (39.5C), **hypotension** (BP 80/60); **tachycardia** (HR 120). PE: toxic-looking; **icteric**; abdominal exam reveals extremely **tender RUQ with hepatomegaly**.

Labs   CBC: **leukocytosis with neutrophilia**. LFTs: **markedly elevated bilirubin, AST, ALT, alkaline phosphatase and GGT**. Blood cultures grew *Escherichia coli*.

Imaging   CT, abdomen: **multiple hepatic abscesses**; distended gallbladder with perihepatic and pericholecystic fluid collections.

Treatment   **Prolonged IV antibiotic therapy**; emergent endoscopic (ERCP) or surgical biliary decompression; surgical **drainage** of the **abscesses** if no response to IV antibiotics.

Discussion   **A pyogenic liver abscess** is a pus-filled cavity within the liver caused by a bacterial infection, typically polymicrobial. The causes of liver abscess include **abdominal infection** such as appendicitis, diverticulitis, or perforated bowel; **sepsis; biliary tract infection**; or **liver trauma** leading to secondary infection. The most common bacteria involved are *E. coli, Klebsiella* **spp.,** *Enterococcus, Staphylococcus* **spp.,** *Streptococcus* **spp.,** and *Bacteroides*. Positive blood cultures are found in about half of patients with a pyogenic liver abscess and sepsis is a life-threatening complication. There is significant mortality even in treated patients and mortality is higher in those with multiple abscesses.

ID/CC A 30-year-old **dairy farm worker** presents with complaints of **fever, headache, cough, pleuritic chest pain**, and malaise.

HPI His work at the dairy involves **milking cows** and **looking after parturient cattle**.

PE VS: fever; tachypnea. PE: mild icterus; bilateral **crackles** on chest auscultation.

Labs CBC: normal WBC count. Mild elevation of serum bilirubin and liver enzymes; greater than fourfold increase in **complement-fixing antibody (against *Coxiella burnetii*)** titer between acute and convalescent sera (IFA technique for early detection of specific IgM Ab is the serodiagnostic method of choice); **negative Weil-Felix reaction**; *C. burnetii* isolated from sputum by inoculation of cultured human fetal diploid fibroblasts.

Imaging CXR: right upper lobe **rounded opacity** that increased in size over a few days and cleared completely with treatment.

Treatment **Doxycycline** is the first-line agent of therapy (erythromycin can also be used).

Discussion Q fever is caused by the rickettsia-like organism *Coxiella burnetii* and produces the clinical picture of primary atypical pneumonia. Q fever differs from the other human rickettsioses in that rash is absent and **transmission** is usually **by the airborne route**. *C. burnetii* localizes in the **mammary glands and uterus of pregnant cattle**, sheep, and goats, in which infection is mild or inapparent; **infected placentas, postpartum discharges, and the feces of these animals** are the **principal sources of contaminated material** in the environment. Humans acquire Q fever by inhaling aerosolized particles from such substances; particularly **at risk** are **dairy and slaughterhouse workers**.

ID/CC A 12-year-old white female is rushed to the emergency room because of **numbness** of the right foot and leg followed by **fever** and **convulsions**. The child **refuses to drink any fluids** (HYDROPHOBIA).

HPI She had been camping 5 weeks ago. When questioned, her mother recalls that one night the child had apparently stepped on **a bat that bit her in the right foot**.

PE VS: no fever. PE: child is **disoriented, hyperventilating**, extremely agitated, and actively moving all four limbs; thus **difficult to restrain**; no meningeal signs; fundus normal; **saliva viscous and foaming**.

Labs LP: lymphocytic pleocytosis with mildly elevated proteins and normal sugar in CSF. **Positive rabies antigen in corneal scrapings**.

Micro Pathology Characteristic **cytoplasmic inclusion bodies** (NEGRI BODIES) in **corneal scrapings** or **Ammon's horn**.

Treatment Supportive; almost always fatal; prevent with vaccine; postexposure prophylaxis with diploid cell vaccine and human rabies immune globulin (HRIG).

Discussion Rabies is a fatal viral disease that is transmitted to humans by the bites of **bats, raccoons**, skunks, foxes, coyotes, dogs, and cats. Rabies virus is an enveloped, single-stranded RNA virus. Rabies has a **long incubation period** (approximately 3 to 8 weeks); death usually results from respiratory failure.

Atlas Link UCV1 M-M2-041

ID/CC	A 27-year-old male **researcher** presents with sudden-onset **fever**, chills, headache, a **skin rash**, and **painful** swelling of multiple limb **joints**.
HPI	Careful history reveals that he was **bitten by a rat** in his laboratory a few days ago; the bite wound has now healed.
PE	VS: **fever**. PE: morbilliform **rash** noted over extremities, particularly the hands and feet; **painful swelling** and restriction of movement noted over **both wrist and knee joints**.
Labs	CBC: leukocytosis. *Streptobacillus moniliformis* isolated from blood and synovial fluid of inflamed joints; agglutinins to *S. moniliformis* demonstrated in significant titers.
Treatment	**Amoxicillin/clavulonic acid** (**doxycycline** can also be used).
Discussion	Rat bite fever, which is caused by *Streptobacillus moniliformis*, is an acute febrile illness that is usually accompanied by a skin rash; **most cases result from the bites of wild or lab rats**, although mice, squirrels, weasels, dogs, and cats may also transmit the disease by bites or scratches. The disease is called **Haverhill fever** when *S. moniliformis* is transmitted by drinking rat-excrement-contaminated milk. Distribution is probably worldwide, with most cases occurring in crowded cities characterized by poor sanitation.

ID/CC A 30-year-old male who lives in the **western part of the United States** presents with **high fever**, shaking **chills**, severe headache, myalgias, and diarrhea.

HPI He reports having had **similar symptoms 10 days ago** that lasted for 4 to 5 days, followed by defervescence accompanied by drenching sweats and marked prostration. He had been **hiking in a tick-infested forest** until about a week before the development of symptoms.

PE VS: **fever**.

Labs **Spirochetes found on thick smears of peripheral blood** obtained during febrile period and **stained with Wright or Giemsa stain**.

Treatment **Doxycycline** is the drug of choice (erythromycin may also be used).

Discussion Relapsing fever is an **acute louse-borne or tick-borne infection** that is caused by blood spirochetes of the genus *Borrelia*; it is characterized by **recurrent febrile episodes separated by asymptomatic intervals**. Unlike other spirochetes, the etiologic agent can readily be detected with Giemsa stain or Wright's stain. *B. recurrentis* is the **cause of louse-borne relapsing fever**, whereas a variety of different species produce the **tick-borne disease**. In the United States, the predominant species are *B. hermsii* and *B. turicatae*. Most patients experience the Jarisch–Herxheimer reaction within the first 2 hours of treatment.

ID/CC	A 6-year-old male presents with fever, intense headache, myalgia, dry cough, and a **rash that began peripherally** (on his wrists and ankles) but now involves the entire body, **including the palms and soles**.
HPI	The child lives in North Carolina and indicates that he was **bitten by an insect** a few weeks ago while playing in the woods near his home.
PE	VS: fever. PE: lethargy; ill appearance; **petechial rash** all over body, including palms and soles.
Labs	CBC: thrombocytopenia; prolonged bleeding and clotting time. Positive Hess capillary test (RUMPEL-LEEDE PHENOMENON); **positive *Proteus* OX19 and OX2 Weil-Felix reaction**; specific antibodies to *Rickettsia rickettsii* with positive complement fixation. UA: proteinuria; hematuria.
Gross Pathology	Hemorrhagic necrosis in brain and kidneys; nodular formation in glia.
Micro Pathology	Inflammatory lymphocytic and plasma cell perivascular infiltration; endothelial edema with abundant rickettsiae; microthrombus formation **with necrotic vasculitis**.
Treatment	**Doxycycline** or **chloramphenicol**.
Discussion	*Rickettsia rickettsii* is the causative organism of Rocky Mountain spotted fever; *Dermacentor*, **a wood tick, is the vector**. The organism's tropism for endothelial cells results in vasculitis, edema, thrombosis, and ischemia. Ironically, Rocky Mountain spotted fever is endemic to the East Coast of the United States.

ROCKY MOUNTAIN SPOTTED FEVER

ID/CC	A **5-month-old** male infant is brought to the pediatric clinic with **wheezing and respiratory difficulty** of 3 hours' duration.
HPI	He has had rhinorrhea, fever, and cough and had been sneezing for 2 days prior to his visit to the clinic.
PE	VS: tachypnea. PE: nasal flaring; mild **central cyanosis**; accessory muscle use during respiration; hyperexpansion of chest; **expiratory and inspiratory wheezes; rhonchi** over both lung fields.
Labs	CBC/PBS: relative lymphocytosis. ABGs: hypoxemia with mild hypercapnia. Normal flora on bacterial culture of sputum; **respiratory syncytial virus (RSV)** demonstrated on viral culture of throat swab.
Imaging	CXR: hyperinflation; segmental atelectasis; interstitial infiltrates.
Treatment	Humidified oxygen; bronchodilators; aerosolized **ribavirin**.
Discussion	RSV is the **most common cause of bronchiolitis in infants** under 2 years of age; other viral causes include parainfluenza, influenza, and adenovirus. Infections typically occur during the fall and winter months. Transmission occurs via close contact with contaminated fomites but can also occur after coughing or sneezing. The majority of infections occur during an RSV epidemic.

INFECTIOUS DISEASE

RSV PNEUMONIA

ID/CC	A 4-month-old girl brought in for a well-child visit is found to be **low in weight and height for her age** and to have **lens opacities** (due to congenital cataracts).
HPI	Her mother had a skin rash and fever during her **first trimester**. The mother states that when the child was born, she too had a **rash** like a "blueberry muffin" and was **jaundiced**.
PE	**Deaf** and **globally retarded**; malnourished; **microcephaly** and bulging anterior fontanelle; **microphthalmia** with unilateral left **cataract**; discrete black, patchy pigmentation found in retina on funduscopic exam; **hepatosplenomegaly; machinery murmur heard at second intercostal space** on left sternal border (due to **patent ductus arteriosus**).
Labs	CBC/PBS: leukopenia; thrombocytopenia. Increased serum bilirubin (both direct and indirect); rubella virus isolated from urine and saliva; markedly increased **IgM specific antibody for rubella**.
Imaging	XR, plain: radiolucent (lytic) bone lesions (metaphyseal).
Treatment	None.
Discussion	Congenital rubella, transmitted in utero, is caused by rubella virus, a single-stranded RNA togavirus. In children and adults it is a transitory and unremarkable disease. If acquired **in utero it has devastating consequences**.

ID/CC	A 10-year-old female Asian immigrant presents with a **low-grade fever** and coryza of 3 days' duration.
HPI	She also complains of arthralgias and a **skin rash that began on her face and spread to her trunk**. Her mother says she cannot remember any details of her vaccination history.
PE	VS: fever. PE: maculopapular rash over face and trunk; **enlarged postauricular, posterior cervical, and occipital lymph nodes**.
Labs	CBC: leukopenia; thrombocytopenia. Rubella virus hemagglutination inhibition test demonstrates **fourfold rise in titer** to 1:32.
Gross Pathology	Erythematous skin rash resembling rubeola measles but lighter in color and more discrete; similar distribution pattern in both.
Treatment	Symptomatic treatment.
Discussion	Rubella (German measles) is caused by a togavirus. Live attenuated rubella virus vaccine (part of MMR) should be given to all infants and to susceptible girls before menarche. The course of illness is self-limiting and mild; in females the major implication is the potential for congenital rubella syndrome. Females with rubella can get **polyarthritis** secondary to immune complex deposition.
Atlas Link	UCV2 IM2-026

RUBELLA (GERMAN MEASLES)

ID/CC	A 14-year-old male who is known to have **sickle cell anemia** presents with throbbing **pain, redness**, and **swelling** of the **right thigh**.
HPI	The patient also complains of fever and chills of 1 week's duration. He has a few **pet turtles** at home.
PE	VS: **fever**; tachycardia. PE: pallor; redness, swelling, and tenderness over right thigh; effusion demonstrated in right knee joint; limitation of range of motion of right knee.
Labs	CBC: leukocytosis; elevated ESR. PBS: irreversible **sickling**; blood culture reveals *Salmonella typhimurium* (most common); organism also isolated from pus aspirated from right femur (diagnostic of **osteomyelitis**).
Imaging	Nuc: **increased uptake in metaphyseal region** of right femur. XR (usually normal during the first 10 days of illness) may reveal changes of bone resorption, detached necrotic cortical bone (SEQUESTRUM), and laminated periosteal new-bone formation (INVOLUCRUM).
Gross Pathology	Dense, pale, sclerotic-appearing area in shaft.
Micro Pathology	Changes include suppurative and ischemic destructive necrosis, fibrosis, and ultimate bone repair.
Treatment	**Parenteral antibiotics**, with **fluoroquinolones** being first-line agents (**third-generation cephalosporins** may also be used).
Discussion	A striking association has been noted between diseases producing hemolysis (e.g., sickle cell anemia, malaria, and bartonellosis) and salmonella infections; elderly patients with impaired host defense mechanisms, those with hepatosplenic schistosomiasis, and AIDS patients are also at increased risk of severe and recurrent salmonella bacteremia. Salmonella osteomyelitis in sickle cell patients presents primarily in young individuals and typically affects long bones. It is believed that the functional asplenic state found in most sickle cell patients contributes to the increased prevalence of salmonella osteomyelitis.

SALMONELLA SEPTICEMIA WITH OSTEOMYELITIS

ID/CC   An Asian refugee **family** comprising a 30-year-old man, his wife, and two schoolchildren present **with complaints of severe itching** over their entire bodies except for their face; the itching increases **during the night**.

HPI   The male family members also report penile and scrotal skin lesions. The family is of **low socioeconomic status** and lives in a single room under **crowded conditions**.

PE   Papulovesicular lesions; **"burrows"** seen in the dorsal interdigital web spaces and flexor aspects of both wrists; lesions also seen around elbows, anterior axillary folds, periumbilical area, lower buttocks, and thighs; **face was spared; scrotal and penile lesions** seen in male members were **nodular** and reddish.

Labs   **Female adult mite** was seen with a hand lens when teased out of her burrow with a needle.

Treatment   Apply **lindane** or **permethrin** (lindane is contraindicated in small children and in pregnant women). All family members must be treated; clothing, linen, and the like should be boiled and washed; fingernails should be trimmed. Use antihistamines or calamine lotion to help control itching.

Discussion   Scabies is caused by infestation with *Sarcoptes scabiei,* **a mite** that bores into the corneal layer of the skin, forming burrows in which it deposits its eggs. The scabies organism does not survive for more than 48 hours away from the host; modes of transmission include close contact with infected individuals, unsanitary conditions, and sexual contact. In adults, certain areas of the body are generally spared, including the face, scalp, and neck.

Atlas Links   ⬚UCV1⬚ M-M2-049   ⬚UCV2⬚ MC-186

INFECTIOUS DISEASE

ID/CC	A 10-year-old white female complains of difficulty swallowing, pain in both ears, and fever of 1 week's duration; she also complains of an extensive skin rash.
HPI	The child is fully immunized and has been well until now.
PE	VS: fever. PE: **extensive erythematous rash** ("GOOSE-PIMPLE SUNBURN") on neck, groin, and axillae; desquamation and **peeling of fingertips**; circumoral pallor; **lines of hyperpigmentation with tiny petechiae** (PASTIA'S SIGN) in antecubital fossae; **bright red lingual papillae superimposed on white coat** ("STRAWBERRY TONGUE"); pharyngitis with exudative tonsillitis; cervical lymphadenopathy; normal eardrums.
Labs	CBC: leukocytosis with neutrophilia. **Group A β-hemolytic** *Streptococcus pyogenes* on throat swab and culture; **elevated ASO titer**.
Gross Pathology	Toxin-induced vasodilation; complications include otitis media, pneumonia, glomerulonephritis, osteomyelitis, and rheumatic fever.
Micro Pathology	Inflammatory polymorphonuclear epidermal infiltrate; interstitial nephritis; lymph node hyperplasia.
Treatment	Penicillin; erythromycin.
Discussion	Scarlet fever is a streptococcal infection that is characterized by **morbilliform rash** due to **hypersensitivity to erythrogenic toxin**.
Atlas Links	⬚ⓊⒸⓋ② MC-187A, MC-187B

ID/CC   A 27-year-old Peace Corps volunteer working in the **Congo** is sent home after developing **fever, sweats, and abdominal pain** that have not responded to antimalarial treatment.

HPI   Five weeks ago, he developed **severe itching and a macular rash** (SWIMMER'S ITCH) after swimming in a nearby pond.

PE   VS: fever. PE: moderate enlargement of liver and spleen; tender abdomen but no peritoneal irritation.

Labs   CBC/PBS: **marked eosinophilia**. Characteristic large parasite **eggs** with **lateral spines** may be found in stool specimen.

Imaging   Sigmoidoscopy: swollen and erythematous mucosa; many small ulcerations. CT/US, abdomen: hepatosplenomegaly; portal vein dilatation.

Gross Pathology   Skin and liver sites of principal lesions in acute stage; eggs may be found in liver, lungs, intestines, pancreas, spleen, urogenital organs, and brain; chronic stage characterized by granuloma formation in bladder and liver (PERIPORTAL FIBROSIS).

Micro Pathology   Granulomatous reaction and fibrosis.

Treatment   Praziquantel.

Discussion   Schistosomiasis is among the most common parasitic diseases in the world; infection with *Schistosoma mansoni* or *S. japonicum* is acquired by **swimming** in **snail-infested ponds** and lakes. Long-standing infection may lead to noncirrhotic portal fibrosis and portal hypertension. Also known as bilharziasis.

Atlas Link   ⬚⬚⬚⬚ M-M2-051

ID/CC A 12-year-old **immigrant from the Middle East** presents with **terminal hematuria**, dysuria, and increased frequency of micturition.

HPI He remembers having played and **bathed in snail-infested streams** while he was in his native country; on one occasion he had developed an **intensely pruritic skin eruption** after bathing in one such stream ("CERCARIAL DERMATITIS").

PE Pallor noted.

Labs UA: **hematuria**; mild proteinuria and sterile **(abacterial) pyuria**. Microscopic exam of urine and rectal biopsy reveals presence of **ellipsoid eggs with a sharp terminal spine** containing a miracidium surrounded by a thick, rigid shell.

Imaging XR: bladder wall calcification.

Treatment **Praziquantel**, metrifonate.

Discussion **Three major species** exist. *Schistosoma mansoni, S. japonicum,* and *S. haematobium* infect humans. *S. mansoni* is found in Africa, the Arabian Peninsula, South America, and parts of the Caribbean; *S. japonicum* is found in Japan, China, and the Philippines; and *S. haematobium* **is found in Africa and the Middle East**. Transmission of schistosomiasis **cannot occur in the United States** because of the absence of the specific freshwater **snail that is an intermediary host**. In *S. haematobium* infection, the principal symptoms are terminal hematuria, dysuria, and frequent urination; **hydronephrosis**, pyelonephritis, and **squamous cell carcinoma of the urinary bladder** may develop as **complications**. In *S. mansoni* **and** *S. japonicum* infection, manifestations may include **fever, malaise, abdominal pain, diarrhea**, or hepatosplenomegaly. Presinusoidal hepatic trapping of eggs and the consequent granulomatous reaction induce **portal hypertension**.

ID/CC	A 36-year-old male executive comes to the emergency room because of the development of **sudden nausea, vomiting, and diarrhea** with **blood and mucus** (dysentery) as well as crampy abdominal pain for 2 days.
HPI	He had just returned from a business trip in **South America**.
PE	VS: low-grade fever. PE: mild dehydration; hyperactive bowel sounds; tender abdomen without definite peritoneal irritation.
Labs	**Leukocytes on stool examination**; *Shigella* isolated on stool culture; on microbiology, organism does not ferment lactose and is **not motile**.
Micro Pathology	*Shigella* enterotoxin acts by activating adenylate cyclase; organism invades intestinal mucosa.
Treatment	Rehydration with antibiotic therapy (ampicillin or TMP-SMX).
Discussion	Shigellosis outbreaks occur primarily in areas with **overcrowding** and **poor hygiene** (fecal-oral transmission); **arthritis, conjunctivitis, and urethritis** (REITER'S SYNDROME) may be complications in HLA-B27-positive individuals. Like *Salmonella*, *Shigella* causes bloody diarrhea by invading the intestinal mucosa, causing intestinal ulceration and inflammation.

ID/CC	A 56-year-old hospitalized male is found to have an abrupt-onset **high-grade fever** with chills a few hours after he underwent nephrolithotomy.
HPI	He was diagnosed with chronic nephrolithiasis with **recurrent UTIs**; a surgery intern also noted **poor urine output**.
PE	VS: fever; tachycardia; **hypotension**; tachypnea. PE: confused and disoriented; hyperventilating; diaphoresis; **hands warm** and pink with rapid capillary refill; pulse bounding; on chest auscultation, air entry found to be bilaterally reduced.
Labs	CBC: **leukocytosis** with left shift; neutrophils contain **toxic granulations, Döhle bodies**, and cytoplasmic vacuoles; band forms > 10%; thrombocytopenia. Prolongation of thrombin time, decreased fibrinogen, and presence of D-dimers (suggesting DIC); raised BUN and creatinine. ABGs: metabolic acidosis (increased anion gap due to lactic acidosis) and hypoxemia (due to **ARDS**). Blood and urine **culture yields** *Escherichia coli*.
Imaging	CXR: evidence of noncardiogenic pulmonary edema (ARDS).
Treatment	**IV antibiotics** (with adequate gram-negative coverage); management of multiorgan failure (azotemia, ARDS, and DIC).
Discussion	Almost any bacterium can cause a bacteremia, including *E. coli* (most common), *Klebsiella, Proteus, Pseudomonas* (associated with antibiotic therapy and burn wounds), *Bacteroides fragilis* (causes of anaerobic septicemias), *Staphylococcus aureus, Streptococcus pneumoniae*, and pediatric septicemia due to *E. coli* and *Streptococcus agalactiae*. Gram-negative bacteria release endotoxins; the release of endotoxin into the circulation leads to the activation of macrophages and monocytes, which in turn release cytokines. These cytokines trigger cascade reactions that lead to the clinical and biochemical manifestations of the sepsis syndrome.
Atlas Links	[UCV1] M-M2-054A, M-M2-054B

ID/CC A 37-year-old **gardener** complains of lumps with **red streaks** on his arm and swelling of the axillary lymph nodes.

HPI Two weeks ago, he **pricked his hand with a thorn** while pruning roses. A **nodule** then formed which subsequently **ulcerated** and filled with pus.

PE Nonpainful nodular lesion on dorsum of hand with ulcer formation and suppuration; **tender, palpable inflammation and hardening of lymph vessels** (LYMPHANGITIS); **swelling, inflammation, and suppuration of lymph nodes** (LYMPHADENITIS); nonulcerated satellite nodules along course of lymphatics.

Labs Cigar-shaped budding cells (*SPOROTHRIX SCHENCKII*) visible in pus; diagnosis confirmed by culture of aspirate of nodule.

Gross Pathology **Nonpainful, soft, ulcerated nodule at inoculation site** (SPOROTRICHOTIC CHANCRE); may extend to deep tissues and bone with osteitis and synovitis.

Micro Pathology Usually area of suppuration with polymorphonuclear infiltrate surrounded by granulomatous reaction of varied intensity with epithelioid and giant cell formation; chlamydospore asteroid bodies present.

Treatment Itraconazole; potassium iodide.

Discussion Also called **"rose gardener's disease,"** sporotrichosis is a fungal infection caused by *Sporothrix schenckii*, a dimorphic fungus that lives on vegetation. It is typically transmitted by a thorn prick and causes localized infection with few systemic manifestations.

Atlas Link [UCVI] M-M2-055

ID/CC	A 7-year-old girl is seen by the embassy doctor in **Nigeria** for abdominal pain, **diarrhea, fever, dry cough**, and marked **dyspnea** of 2 weeks' duration.
HPI	She is the daughter of an American diplomat working in Nigeria. Despite her parent's admonitions, she frequently **walks barefoot**.
PE	VS: fever. PE: moderate respiratory distress; no cyanosis; no clubbing; coarse, crepitant rales and **wheezing** heard over both lung fields; mild abdominal tenderness.
Labs	CBC/PBS: **marked eosinophilia**. Typical **motile rhabditiform larvae** on sputum exam as well as in freshly passed stool; positive filarial complement fixation test.
Imaging	CXR: **bilateral, transient migratory infiltrates**.
Gross Pathology	Pneumonitis produced by migration of larvae through respiratory tract.
Treatment	**Ivermectin, thiabendazole**.
Discussion	Strongyloidiasis is seen in the presence of **poor hygiene** and in tropical countries. Larvae penetrate the skin, gaining entrance to the venous system and to the lungs, and then ascend to enter the GI tract.
Atlas Link	UCV1 M-M2-056

STRONGYLOIDIASIS

ID/CC	A 54-year-old white female complains of **spiking fever**, chills, **loss of appetite**, several bouts of diarrhea, and **right upper quadrant pain**.
HPI	**Ten days ago** she underwent an apparently uncomplicated emergency **surgery for suppurative cholecystitis** and was subsequently discharged and sent home.
PE	VS: fever. PE: pallor; slight icterus; **pain on percussion of right costal region**; well-healed surgical wound with no evidence of infection; liver not palpable; crepitant rales on right lung base.
Labs	CBC: **elevated WBC count (17,000) with predominance of neutrophils**.
Imaging	CXR: elevated right hemidiaphragm; slight right pleural effusion. US/CT: **complex fluid collection below diaphragm**.
Treatment	Percutaneous drainage under ultrasonic or fluoroscopic guidance followed by regular blood and radiologic exams; surgical exploration and drainage.
Discussion	Subdiaphragmatic abscess most commonly occurs after abdominal surgery, mainly with septic, emergency procedures; it typically presents 1 week or more postoperatively.

SUBDIAPHRAGMATIC ABSCESS

ID/CC	A 6-week-old male, the son of a **prostitute**, is brought to the family doctor because of persistent, sometimes **bloody mucopurulent nasal discharge, anal ulcers**, and a generalized **rash**.
HPI	The child was delivered at home, and the mother did not receive any prenatal care.
PE	Weak-looking, **icteric** infant with hoarse cry; does not move right limb **(pseudoparalysis)**; bloody purulent discharge evident at nares; generalized lymphadenopathy; hepatosplenomegaly; **maculopapular rash** with desquamation on back and buttocks; **bullae on hands and feet**.
Labs	CBC: anemia. **VDRL** in both mother and child **positive**; direct hyperbilirubinemia; negative Coombs' test; *Treponema pallidum* seen on nasal exudate and anal ulcers.
Imaging	XR, plain: periostitis of long bones; bilateral moth-eaten lesions; focal defect in proximal tibial epiphysis with increased density of epiphyseal line (WIMBERGER'S SIGN).
Gross Pathology	Pathologic features seen if neonatal disease is left untreated include syphilitic chondritis and rhinitis (causes **saddle-nose deformity**), pathologic fractures, **bowing of the tibia** (SABER SHIN), **V-shaped incisors** (HUTCHINSON'S TEETH), multicuspid molars (MULBERRY MOLARS), interstitial keratitis, and deafness.
Treatment	**Penicillin**.
Discussion	*Treponema pallidum* is a spirochete; in utero vertical transmission occurs from an infected mother to the fetus. Congenital syphilis occurs maximally during 16 to 36 weeks of gestation and may be the cause of stillbirth. It is preventable if the mother has received adequate treatment.

ID/CC	An 18-year-old white male presents with a **painless ulcer** on his **penis**.
HPI	He admits to having had **unprotected intercourse** with a prostitute 3 weeks ago.
PE	**Painless, single, rounded, firm papule with well-defined margins on dorsal aspect of glans penis that ulcerates** ("HARD CHANCRE."); nontender, rubbery bilateral inguinal lymphadenopathy.
Labs	Treponemes on **dark-field examination** of exudate from chancre; VDRL positive; **FTA-ABS positive**; ELISA for HIV negative.
Gross Pathology	A 1.2-cm ulcerated papule with rolled edges and induration; regional lymphadenopathy.
Micro Pathology	Capillary dilatation with plasma cell, PMN, and macrophage infiltration; fibroblastic reaction.
Treatment	**Benzathine penicillin G** IM, 2.4 MU single dose.
Discussion	An STD caused by *Treponema pallidum*, a spirochete, primary syphilis is characterized by the appearance of a painless chancre in the area of inoculation. If left untreated, secondary and tertiary syphilis may ensue. Other STDs, such as AIDS, are more prevalent in patients with syphilis.
Atlas Link	ⅢⅭⅤ❷ Z-M2-059

INFECTIOUS DISEASE

SYPHILIS—PRIMARY

ID/CC A 23-year-old female presents with a **nonpruritic skin eruption, hair loss**, and generalized fatigue and weakness.

HPI She admits to having had **multiple sexual partners** and **unprotected sex**. She has had two spontaneous abortions.

PE Extensive **raised, copper-colored, maculopapular, desquamative rash on palms and soles**; generalized nontender **lymphadenopathy** with hepatosplenomegaly; large, pale, **coalescent, flat-topped papules and plaques** in groin (CONDYLOMATA LATA); dull, erythematous **mucous patches in mouth**; hair loss (ALOPECIA) in tail of eyebrows.

Labs Skin lesions, mucous patches in mouth, and condylomata lata positive for **treponemes; positive VDRL; positive FTA-ABS**; ELISA negative for HIV; CSF VDRL negative.

Treatment IM benzathine **penicillin G**.

Discussion **Sexual partners must be treated**.

Atlas Links ⬛UCV2 IM2-027A, IM2-027B

ID/CC	A 54-year-old man presents with **ataxia, mental status changes**, grossly **deformed ankle joints**, and **shooting pains** in his extremities.
HPI	He remembers having had a "boil" on his penis (PRIMARY SYPHILITIC CHANCRE) many years ago that went away by itself. He also recalls having had a scaling rash on the soles of his feet and the palms of his hands (due to secondary syphilis) some time ago.
PE	Painless **subcutaneous granulomatous nodules** (GUMMAS); **reduced joint position and vibration sense in both lower extremities** (due to bilateral dorsal column destruction); loss of deep tendon reflexes in both lower limbs; loss of pain sensation and **deformed ankle and knee joints with effusion** (CHARCOT'S NEUROPATHIC ARTHROPATHY); **broad-based gait**; positive Romberg's sign (due to sensory ataxia); **pupillary light reflex lost but accommodation reflex retained** (ARGYLL ROBERTSON PUPILS).
Labs	Positive VDRL and *Treponema pallidum* hemagglutination assay (TP-HA). **LP: pleocytosis and increased proteins in CSF**; VDRL positive. Normal blood glucose levels.
Imaging	CXR: **"tree-bark calcification" of ascending aorta.**
Gross Pathology	Obliterative endarteritis and meningoencephalitis.
Micro Pathology	Proliferation of microglia; demyelinization and axonal loss in dorsal roots and columns.
Treatment	Penicillin.
Discussion	**Tabes dorsalis** usually develops 15 to 20 years after initial infection. There may also be visceral involvement (can cause neurogenic bladder).
Atlas Link	ⓊⒸⓋ② IM2-028

81 **SYPHILIS—TERTIARY (TABES DORSALIS)**

ID/CC A 12-year-old white male presents with **stiffness of the jaw** and neck along with inability to swallow.

HPI Twelve days ago he stepped on a **rusty nail**, which produced a small **puncture wound**; the area is now red, hard, and swollen with pus. He has been experiencing tingling sensations and spasms in his calf muscles. He has not received any immunizations within the past 10 years.

PE **Jaw muscle rigidity** (TRISMUS); **facial muscle spasm** (RISUS SARDONICUS); **dysphagia; neck rigidity**; normal deep tendon reflexes; profuse sweating; patient alert, apprehensive, restless, and hyperactive during PE; loud noise elicits **painful spasms** of face, neck, abdomen, and back, the latter producing **opisthotonos**.

Labs CBC, CSF, blood chemistries normal.

Gross Pathology There may be fractures of ribs or vertebrae with sustained spasms.

Treatment **Surgical debridement of wound**; tetanus immune globulin intra-muscularly or intrathecally; diazepam; phenobarbital; tetanus toxoid; penicillin IV.

Discussion Tetanus is caused by **tetanospasmin**, a neurotoxin produced by *Clostridium tetani*, an obligate anaerobic, spore-forming, gram-positive rod; the toxin blocks the release of the inhibitory neu-rotransmitter glycine in the anterior horn cells. Tetanus often occurs in IV drug abusers; neonates of nonimmunized mothers may become infected through the **umbilical cord stump**. The disease may occur even **years** after injury or infection and may also involve the autonomic nervous system (arrhythmias, high/low blood pressure).

Atlas Link UCV1 M-M2-062

ID/CC A 15-day-old **infant** is brought by his mother to the pediatric emergency room in a state of marked **muscle rigidity and spasm**.

HPI The mother is illiterate and did **not receive any prenatal care**; the delivery was conducted at home and, according to her, was uneventful and full term. The child did **not receive any immunizations**; directed questioning reveals that he has been crying excessively for the past 2 weeks and has not been feeding normally.

PE Extremely ill-looking infant in a state of **generalized rigidity and opisthotonus**; on slightest touch or noise, spasm worsens and he develops a stridor and becomes cyanosed.

Labs Diagnosis is largely clinical; **culture of umbilical stump yields *Clostridium tetani*.**

Treatment **Ventilatory assistance; supportive** management; maintenance of nutritional, fluid, and electrolyte balance; **tetanus antitoxin**; control of tetanic spasms with diazepam.

Discussion Tetanus neonatorum accounts for a considerable proportion of infant deaths in developing countries, primarily owing to the **lack of availability of good prenatal care** (no tetanus immunization); untrained birth attendants in rural areas use **contaminated** material to cut or anoint the **umbilical cord**. Tetanus is caused by *Clostridium tetani*, a gram-positive, motile, nonencapsulated, anaerobic, spore-bearing bacillus; its effects are mediated through production of a powerful **neurotoxin (tetanospasmin)**. The toxin acts principally on the spinal cord, altering normal control of the reflex arc by suppressing the inhibition regularly mediated by the internuncial neurons.

ID/CC	A 40-year-old male who recently went **hiking in a forest** in the **western United States** presents with **symmetric weakness** of the lower extremities that has now progressed over the past few days to involve the trunk and the upper arms.
HPI	The patient does not report any sensory symptoms.
PE	Higher mental functions intact; **symmetric flaccid paralysis** with an **ascending pattern** of spread noted; **no sensory loss** demonstrated; on careful examination of hairy areas of the body, a **tick** was found **embedded in the scalp**.
Labs	LP: CSF normal. EMG: nerve conduction velocity and compound muscle action potentials decreased.
Treatment	Tick was **detached without being squeezed**, and this led to **resolution of symptoms** over the next few days.
Discussion	Feeding ticks may elaborate a **neurotoxin** that causes tick paralysis; symmetric weakness of the lower extremities progresses to an **ascending flaccid paralysis** over several hours to days, although the sensorium remains clear and sensory function is normal.

ID/CC   A 40-year-old male diagnosed with **AIDS** presents with a **severe headache**.

HPI   He suffered a grand mal seizure 2 hours before his arrival in the emergency room. He denies any history of seizures and adds that he has many pets, including **cats**.

PE   **Generalized lymphadenopathy**; bilateral **papilledema**; left-sided hemiparesis with hyperactive deep tendon reflexes on left side; positive Babinski's sign on left side.

Labs   Positive indirect fluorescent antibody test for toxoplasmosis; positive Sabin-Feldman dye test.

Imaging   MR/CT, head: single or multiple rounded **mass lesions with ring or nodular enhancement**.

Gross Pathology   Large brain abscesses with concomitant focal neurologic abnormalities, seizures, or altered mental status.

Micro Pathology   Parasites appear in tissue as tachyzoites or encysted bradyzoites; aggregates of nonencapsulated organisms constitute pseudocysts.

Treatment   Pyrimethamine; sulfadiazine.

Discussion   The **definitive host** of *Toxoplasma gondii* is the domestic **cat**. The intermediate hosts are many and varied, including humans. Toxoplasmosis is also transmitted by ingestion of raw or undercooked meat.

Atlas Links   UCV1 M-M2-065   UCV2 MC-191

TOXOPLASMOSIS

ID/CC	A 50-year-old man presents with generalized **myalgia** and a persistent **low-grade fever**.
HPI	In addition, the patient recalled having severe **abdominal pain and diarrhea several weeks ago**. The patient worked in a **pig slaughterhouse** for many years.
PE	VS: fever. PE: periorbital and facial edema; tenderness over calf, thigh, and shoulder muscles; conjunctival and splinter hemorrhages; no neurologic deficit seen.
Labs	CBC: **eosinophilia**. Normal ESR; **elevated serum CPK, LDH, and AST**; latex agglutination test positive for *Trichinella*.
Gross Pathology	Facial, neck, biceps, lower back, and diaphragm most frequently affected muscles.
Micro Pathology	Biopsy of sternocleidomastoid muscle reveals cysts of *Trichinella spiralis*.
Treatment	Albendazole; mebendazole; high-dose corticosteroids.
Discussion	The organism causing trichinosis, *Trichinella spiralis*, can be transmitted when **raw or undercooked pork** is ingested. The larvae develop only in **striated muscle cells**.
Atlas Link	UCV1 M-M2-066

ID/CC	A **6-year-old male** is brought to the ER in a **delirious state** with fever and marked **dyspnea** that have rapidly progressed over the past 2 days.
HPI	His **mother**, an **Asian immigrant**, was diagnosed and treated for **pulmonary tuberculosis** a few months ago. He has had a low-grade **fever**, cough, **malaise**, and **night sweats** for the past 2 months. The child has not received prophylactic isoniazid or BCG vaccination.
PE	VS: fever; tachycardia; marked tachypnea; hypotension. PE: toxic and stuporous; pallor; **central cyanosis**; extensive rales and rhonchi bilaterally; hepatosplenomegaly; lymphadenopathy; funduscopy reveals **choroidal tubercles**.
Labs	CBC: **lymphocytosis**; normochromic, normocytic anemia. **Increased ESR; Mantoux skin test negative** (false negative may occur during incubation and with severe disease); staining and culture of transbronchial and bone marrow biopsy specimens reveal presence of *Mycobacterium tuberculosis*; PCR for tuberculosis positive; ELISA for HIV negative.
Imaging	CXR: soft, **uniformly distributed fine nodules throughout both lung fields** (MILIARY MOTTLING).
Gross Pathology	Myriad 1- to 2-mm **granulomas** demonstrable in lungs, liver, and bone marrow biopsy specimens.
Micro Pathology	**Granulomas** with **central caseous necrosis** surrounded by epithelial cells, Langerhan's cells, lymphocytes, plasma cells, and fibroblasts in affected tissues.
Treatment	**Multidrug antitubercular therapy** with isoniazid, rifampicin, pyrazinamide, and ethambutol or streptomycin; steroids may be indicated.
Discussion	Miliary tuberculosis results from **widespread hematogenous dissemination** and often presents with a perplexing fever, dyspnea, anemia, and splenomegaly; the disease is **more fulminant in children** than in adults.
Atlas Link	UCVI PG-M2-067

ID/CC	A 14-year-old male immigrant complains of malaise, **weight loss, fever, and night sweats** of 6 weeks' duration; he also has a mild cough that began to produce **bloody sputum** 3 days prior to his admission.
HPI	The patient's **mother** has been diagnosed with pulmonary **tuberculosis** and is currently receiving treatment for it.
PE	VS: mild fever. PE: **malnourished**; low height and weight for age; bronchial breath sounds with crepitant rales heard over right supramammary area.
Labs	CBC/PBS: normocytic, normochromic anemia; WBC count normal with relative **lymphocytosis. Increased ESR**; sputum stained with ZN stain **positive for acid-fast bacilli**; positive radiometric culture for *Mycobacterium tuberculosis*; positive ELISA for TB; positive **intradermal tuberculin injection** (MANTOUX TEST).
Imaging	CXR: small cavity with streaky infiltrates in right upper lobe; hilar lymphadenopathy; calcified lung lesion (GHON'S LESION); Ghon's lesion and calcified lymph node (RANKE COMPLEX).
Gross Pathology	**Primary tuberculosis** usually consists of **lesions in lower lung lobes** and in subpleural locations; cavitation rare; **secondary TB** or reinfection characterized by cavitary lesions usually located in **apical regions**.
Micro Pathology	Multinucleated epithelioid **Langerhan's cells** surround core of **caseating necrosis** in lung parenchyma, producing fibroblastic reaction at periphery with lymphocytic infiltration and proliferation (TUBERCLE).
Treatment	Multiple drug therapy with isoniazid (INH), rifampin, ethambutol, pyrazinamide, and/or streptomycin.
Discussion	Pulmonary tuberculosis is caused by *Mycobacterium tuberculosis*, an acid-fast, gram-positive aerobic bacillus. An **increasing incidence in AIDS patients** has been observed; drug resistance is becoming common.
Atlas Links	UCV1 M-M2-068A, M-M2-068B, M-M2-068C, PG-M2-068A, PG-M2-068B

ID/CC A 12-year-old white male is brought to his pediatrician because of an **ulcer** on his right wrist together with **swelling of the lymph nodes** in the right axillae with **suppuration**.

HPI He had just returned from summer camp and, upon questioning, admits to having played with **rabbits** at the camp's breeding grounds. He has been suffering from **fever**, headache, and muscle aches for almost a week.

PE VS: fever. PE: indurated erythematous nodule with ulcer formation on right wrist; right axillary adenopathy with pus formation; lymphangitis; mild splenomegaly; scattered rales in both lung bases.

Labs CBC: **normal WBC count. Increased ESR**; elevated C-reactive protein; positive agglutination test; *Francisella tularensis* on direct fluorescent antibody staining of material from ulcer.

Imaging CXR: bilateral basilar interstitial infiltrates.

Gross Pathology Enlarged, indurated lymph nodes with necrosis and suppuration; skin nodule at site of inoculation with ulcer formation.

Micro Pathology Necrosis and suppuration of lymph nodes; pulmonary and disseminated lesions; **granulomatous nodules** with central caseating necrosis.

Treatment Streptomycin and gentamicin.

Discussion Tularemia is an acute zoonosis caused by *Francisella tularensis*, a nonmotile, aerobic, gram-negative bacillus; it is transmitted through contact with rabbits, squirrels, or other rodents or tick bites. It may be ulceroglandular, tonsillar, oculoglandular, pneumonitic, or typhoidal.

ID/CC A 27-year-old male is admitted to the hospital for evaluation of **increasing fever** of unknown origin along with malaise, headache, sore throat, cough, and **constipation**.

HPI He visited Southeast Asia 3 weeks ago but did not receive any prior vaccinations.

PE VS: **bradycardia**; fever; **fever charting reveals "stepladder" pattern**. PE: mild hepatosplenomegaly; faint **erythematous macules seen over trunk** ("ROSE SPOTS").

Labs CBC: neutropenia with relative lymphocytosis. **Widal's test positive in significant titers**; blood and stool cultures reveal *Salmonella typhi*.

Gross Pathology **Infection of Peyer's patches** in terminal ileum leads to necrosis of underlying mucosa, producing longitudinal oval ulcerations.

Micro Pathology Ulcers bordered by mononuclear cells; typhoid nodules with lymphocytes and macrophages may be present in liver, spleen, and lymph nodes.

Treatment Ciprofloxacin is curative.

Discussion Because infection is acquired from contaminated food or water, typhoid vaccine is recommended for all those traveling to areas that have had typhoid epidemics. Three vaccines are available: the parenteral vaccine containing the capsular polysaccharide and the oral vaccine containing live attenuated organisms are more effective than the parenteral vaccine containing whole killed organisms. *S. typhi* is transmitted only by humans, whereas all other *Salmonella* species have an animal as well as a human reservoir.

Atlas Link UCV2 IM2-030

ID/CC	A 19-year-old male goes to his health clinic complaining of **painful urination and discharge**.
HPI	The patient had **casual sex with a classmate** while at a party **2 weeks ago**. He has had no previous STDs.
PE	Watery yellowish-green discharge from meatus; no penile ulcerations or inguinal lymphadenopathy.
Labs	**Numerous neutrophils but no bacteria** on Gram stain of discharge; **positive** direct immunofluorescence using mono-clonal **antibody against *Chlamydia***; routine bacterial cultures, including Thayer-Martin, do not show growth.
Treatment	Tetracycline; **doxycycline**; azithromycin; treat both patient and sexual partner.
Discussion	The most common cause of nongonococcal urethritis is *Chlamydia trachomatis*; less frequently it is caused by *Ureaplasma urealyticum*. It is frequently coincident with gonococcal urethritis.
Atlas Link	UCV1 M-M2-071

URETHRITIS—NONGONOCOCCAL

ID/CC	A 25-year-old **sexually active female** complains of **burning on urination**.
HPI	She also complains of pain in the lower abdomen and **increased frequency of urination**.
PE	Mild suprapubic tenderness.
Labs	UA: mild proteinuria; hematuria; WBCs but no casts seen. Urine culture reveals **> 100,000 *Escherichia coli*** organisms present.
Gross Pathology	Infection ascends the urinary tract (urethritis, cystitis, pyelonephritis); mucosal hyperemia and edema.
Micro Pathology	Urothelial hyperplasia and metaplasia.
Treatment	Ciprofloxacin.
Discussion	Eighty percent of UTIs are caused by *E. coli*; *Staphylococcus saprophyticus* is the second most common cause. Other causes, in order of frequency, are *Proteus, Klebsiella, Enterobacter, Serratia, Pseudomonas,* and *Enterococcus*; *Chlamydia* and *Neisseria* are also causes of urethritis. Risk factors include female gender, sexual activity, pregnancy, obstruction, bladder dysfunction, vesicoureteral reflux, and catheterization.

ID/CC	A 25-year-old **sexually active woman** presents with **burning during micturition** (DYSURIA), increased frequency and urgency of micturition, and low-grade fever.
HPI	She is otherwise in perfect health.
PE	VS: fever.
Labs	UA: abundant WBCs; mild proteinuria but no casts; staining of sediment reveals presence of gram-positive cocci. Urine culture isolates **coagulase-negative *Staphylococcus saprophyticus*.**
Treatment	Antibiotics (ampicillin, cotrimoxazole, or ciprofloxacin).
Discussion	Enterobacteriaceae such as *Escherichia coli*, *Klebsiella* species, and *Proteus* and *Pseudomonas* species are the most common organisms causing UTI. After *E. coli*, *Staphylococcus saprophyticus* is the most common cause of primary nonobstructive UTI in sexually active young women.

UTI WITH *STAPHYLOCOCCUS SAPROPHYTICUS*

ID/CC	A 5-year-old male presents with malaise, anorexia, fever, and a **pruritic rash on his scalp**, face, and trunk.
HPI	He also complains of a headache. Six of his **classmates** recently missed school because of **similar symptoms**.
PE	VS: fever (39°C). PE: skin lesions consist of **macules, papules, vesicles, pustules, and scabs, all present at same time**, predominantly over trunk, face, and scalp.
Labs	Multinucleated giant cells on scraping samples from vesicles. CBC: **leukopenia**.
Gross Pathology	Macular, papular, vesicular, and pustular rash with scab formation; characteristically, all lesions present at same time (vs. variola); **lesions appear in crops** every 3 to 5 days; myocarditis and pneumonitis may be present.
Micro Pathology	Intranuclear, acidophilic inclusion bodies (LIPSCHÜTZ BODIES) in epithelial cells with clear halo around them and multinucleated giant cells on histologic exam of skin lesions (on **Tzanck smear**).
Treatment	Acetaminophen; antihistamines and calamine lotion; hygienic measures, including isolation.
Discussion	A highly contagious dermotropic viral disease caused by varicella-zoster virus, a DNA herpesvirus, chickenpox is transmitted by respiratory aerosol or by direct contact. Complications include secondary bacterial infection of the skin and pneumonia; high-risk individuals may be protected passively with immunoglobulin and/or acyclovir.
Atlas Links	UCV1 M-M2-074 UCV2 PED-035

ID/CC	An 8-year-old male is brought to a physician with complaints of **impairment of vision** in the left eye, **urticarial skin rashes**, and ill-defined muscle aches.
HPI	The child's mother has caught the child eating dirt or soil on many occasions (PICA). The family also has a **pet dog** at home.
PE	**Rounded swelling near the optic disk** seen on fundus exam of left eye; **urticarial wheals** observed on extremities and trunk; mild **hepatosplenomegaly** noted.
Labs	Leukocytosis with marked **eosinophilia**; enzyme immunoassay using extracts of excretory-secretory products of *Toxocara canis* **larvae** positive.
Micro Pathology	Biopsy of liver reveals larvae with granuloma and eosinophilic infiltration.
Treatment	**Diethylcarbamazine; albendazole** or **mebendazole**; steroids to control symptomatic inflammatory response; laser photocoagulation of visible ocular larvae.
Discussion	When the nondefinitive human host is infected with parasites that normally infect animals, the parasites do not mature completely, but the larvae introduced persist and induce an inflammatory reaction. The syndrome of **visceral larva migrans** develops when nematode larvae of animal parasites (**mostly cat or dog ascarids** such as *Toxocara canis*) migrate in human tissues; the syndrome of **cutaneous larva migrans** (creeping eruption) develops when the larvae of various parasites (including the **dog or cat hookworm** *Ancylostoma braziliense*) penetrate human skin and form pruritic, serpiginous cutaneous lesions along the migratory tracts of the larvae.

VISCERAL LARVA MIGRANS

ID/CC A 2-year-old female is brought to the emergency room because of **paroxysms** and multiple **coughs** in a single expiration, followed by a high-pitched **inspiratory whistle or whoop**.

HPI For the past 2 weeks she has had a runny nose, low-grade fever, muscle pains, and headache. Her **immunization schedule is incomplete**.

PE VS: fever. PE: child apprehensive and becomes cyanotic during cough paroxysm; thick green mucus expelled with cough; conjunctival injection.

Labs CBC: **marked leukocytosis with lymphocytosis**. *Bordetella pertussis* on fluorescent antibody staining of nasopharyngeal secretions; diagnosis confirmed by culture on Bordet-Gengou medium.

Gross Pathology Small conjunctival and brain hemorrhages may appear during paroxysms; bronchiectasis may also be a complication.

Micro Pathology Signs of acute inflammation in upper respiratory tract mucosa, with erythema, petechiae, polymorphonuclear infiltrate, and necrosis.

Treatment Largely supportive; **erythromycin**.

Discussion A bacterial infection of the upper respiratory tract caused by *Bordetella pertussis*, a gram-negative coccobacillus, whooping cough is transmitted by droplets and comprises three stages: prodromal (catarrhal), paroxysmal (coughing), and convalescent. It is largely preventable with universally administered diphtheria toxoid, tetanus toxoid, and pertussis a cellular (DTP) vaccine. Pertussis toxin is a heat-labile exotoxin in which ADP ribosylates the inhibitory G protein, thus inactivating it and leading to constant activation of adenylate cyclase and increased cAMP. The remarkable lymphocytosis is due to pertussis toxin inhibiting chemokine receptors. As a result, lymphocytes are unable to leave the blood stream.

ID/CC   A **10-year-old child** who lives in **tropical Africa** presents with **multiple papillomatous skin lesions and pain in both legs**.

HPI   The **first lesion** had appeared on the leg as a **small indurated papule that ulcerated** into a granulomatous papilloma.

PE   **Multiple papillomatous skin lesions** seen, especially in intertriginous areas; lesions were painless and exuding a serous fluid; **painful hyperkeratotic lesions** seen on palms and soles; both **tibia were tender** to palpation.

Labs   **Dark-field microscopic examination** of exudate from lesions established the diagnosis by revealing organisms with the **characteristic morphology and rotational motion of pathogenic treponemes**; nontreponemal serologic tests (i.e., VDRL and RPR tests) and treponemal tests (i.e., FTA-ABS test) were positive.

Imaging   XR, legs: evidence of **periostitis of the tibia**.

Treatment   Long-acting intramuscular **benzathine penicillin G** is the treatment of choice.

Discussion   Yaws, the most common of the nonvenereal treponematoses, is a chronic infection of skin and bones caused by *Treponema pertenue*. Yaws occurs in tropical areas of Africa, Asia, and Central and South America; it is principally a disease of childhood, and initial infection occurs between 5 and 15 years of age. Transmission is by direct contact with infected skin lesions containing treponemes and is fostered by conditions of overcrowding and poor hygiene. The disease may occur in three stages: primary, secondary, and tertiary. Only lesions of primary and secondary yaws are infectious.

ID/CC	A 24-year-old white South American male develops sudden **high fever**, chills, generalized aches and pains, retro-orbital headache, nausea, and vomiting.
HPI	He gradually improves, but the fever returns 4 days later along with a **yellowing of his skin and eyes** and an episode of fainting and abundant **coffee-ground emesis**.
PE	VS: fever (39°C); hypotension (BP 90/60). PE: **jaundice**; petechiae on lower legs; swollen, bleeding gums; cardiomegaly; hepatomegaly.
Labs	CBC: leukopenia. UA: oliguria; **albuminuria**; hematuria.
Gross Pathology	Normal-sized liver with yellowish hue and petechiae; pale, swollen kidneys.
Micro Pathology	Characteristic **midzonal lobular necrosis**, fatty accumulation, and eosinophilic intracytoplasmic Councilman bodies on liver biopsy; hyperplasia of endothelial cells surrounding lymphoid follicles of spleen; **severe renal tubular damage** with epithelial fatty degeneration and necrosis.
Treatment	Symptomatic; prevention with mosquito control and live viral vaccination.
Discussion	Yellow fever is a viral hemorrhagic fever that is caused by a flavivirus transmitted by *Aedes* **mosquitoes**; it is preventable by a vaccine, which is required prior to travel to certain countries. It is associated with a mortality rate of 5% to 10%, but most cases are self-limiting and mild. It is similar to malaria but does not recur.

ID/CC   A **neonate died** shortly after birth.

HPI   Review of the medical record reveals history of **refusal to feed**, an extensive **maculopapular skin rash** on his legs and trunk, **respiratory distress**, diarrhea, and seizures shortly after birth.

Discussion   Neonatal listeriosis may occur early or late in neonatal life. Infants may be acutely ill at birth and may die within hours as a result of disseminated listeriosis, which is also called **granulomatosis infantiseptica**. This condition is characterized by **hepatosplenomegaly, thrombocytopenia**, generalized **skin papules**, whitish pharyngeal patches, and **pneumonia**. Commonly, a stained smear of meconium will reveal **gram-positive bacilli**, suggesting the diagnosis.

Atlas Link   UCV1 PG-M2-079

LISTERIA MENINGITIS IN THE NEWBORN

ID/CC A 25-year-old woman visits her family physician because of marked **burning pain while urinating** (DYSURIA), **increased frequency of urination with small amounts of urine** (POLLAKIURIA), and passage of a few drops of **blood-stained** debris at the end of urination (HEMATURIA).

HPI She got married 2 weeks ago and has **just returned from her honeymoon**.

PE VS: no fever; BP normal. PE: no edema; no costovertebral angle tenderness; moderate suprapubic tenderness with **urgency**.

Labs UA: urine collected in two glasses; second glass more turbid and blood-stained; urine sediment reveals RBCs and WBCs; **no RBC or WBC casts**; Gram stain of urine sediment reveals **gram-negative bacilli**; *Escherichia coli* in significant colony count (> 100,000) on urine culture.

Treatment Oral antibiotics (Bactrim, fluoroquinolone); adequate hydration.

Discussion *E. coli* is the most common pathogen; *Proteus, Klebsiella, Staphylococcus saprophyticus*, and *Enterococcus* are other common bacteria causing cystitis. Hemorrhagic cystitis may result from adenoviral infection.

ID/CC	A **28-year-old man** comes to the ER with gradually worsening and now severe **scrotal swelling** and pain radiating to the inguinal area.
HPI	The patient has no significant medical history. He reports pain on urination (due to concomitant urethritis) and notes that he is sexually active with multiple partners. He also notes that the pain is greater on standing and walking and is relieved by rest and elevation of the legs.
PE	VS: normal. PE: **scrotal edema** and erythema; **right epididymis enlarged and tender**; induration present; **elevation** of scrotal contents **relieves pain** (PREHN'S SIGN).
Labs	UA: pyuria. Culture negative; biopsy of epididymis inoculated into cell cultures grows *Chlamydia trachomatis*; immunofluorescence reveals **subtype D.**
Imaging	US: hypoechoic, enlarged epididymis with hypervascularity.
Gross Pathology	Nonspecific inflammation characterized by congestion and edema.
Micro Pathology	Early stage of the infection is limited to the interstitial connective tissue with white cell infiltration.
Treatment	Antibiotics like doxycycline, minocycline for chlamydia. Course of ofloxacin covers all possibilities of causative organisms.
Discussion	Differentiate epididymitis from testicular torsion and tumor (scrotal ultrasonography or isotopic flow study may be needed for differentiating). Transmitted sexually in young adults and most often **caused by *Chlamydia trachomatis* subtypes D through K** and *Neisseria gonorrhoeae*. In those older than 40, *Escherichia coli* and *Pseudomonas* cause most infections. If associated with rectal intercourse, it may be due to Enterobacteriaceae.

ID/CC	A 15-year-old male presents with **painful bilateral swelling of the parotid glands**, left-sided scrotal pain, and fever.
HPI	Nothing in the patient's history suggests that he had childhood mumps. He has not received a measles-mumps-rubella (MMR) vaccination.
PE	VS: fever. PE: bilateral parotid gland enlargement with obliteration of mandibular hollow; hyperemia and edema of Stensen's duct (parotid duct) orifice; retroauricular lymphadenopathy; left-sided scrotal and **testicular swelling with tenderness**.
Labs	CBC: leukopenia with **lymphocytosis; hyperamylasemia**. Positive complement fixation antibodies; positive serologic enzyme immunoassay (EIA) for mumps antibody (repeat test after 1 week to demonstrate a fourfold rise).
Imaging	US, scrotum: increased color flow and edema.
Gross Pathology	Enlarged, edematous testicle.
Micro Pathology	Parotid glands show perivascular mononuclear, lymphocytic, and plasma cell infiltrate with necrosis; ductal obstruction and edema; testicular interstitial edema; perivascular cerebral lymphocytic cuffing.
Treatment	Scrotal support; analgesics, ice packs; corticosteroids.
Discussion	Orchitis may be caused by bacterial infections such as *Escherichia coli* and other enterobacteria; viral infections such as **mumps**; STDs such as *Chlamydia* species or gonorrhea; or pathogens such as *Mycobacterium tuberculosis*. Mumps orchitis may give rise to sterility if bilateral.
Atlas Link	UCV1 PG-M2-082

ID/CC	A **10-year-old child** presents with complaints of acute-onset voiding of **tea-colored urine** and **reduced urinary output**.
HPI	The child was treated 1 week ago for **streptococcal pyoderma** that was confirmed by culture. He also complains of puffiness around the eyes and mild swelling of both feet.
PE	VS: **hypertension** (BP 140/96); fever; tachycardia. PE: periorbital swelling; mild pitting **pedal edema**; no ascites or kidney mass palpable.
Labs	CBC: mild leukocytosis. Elevated BUN and creatinine; **elevated ASO titer**; serum cryoglobulins present. UA: **RBC casts; proteinuria. C3 levels reduced** in blood.
Gross Pathology	Smooth, reddish-brown cortical surface with numerous petechial hemorrhages.
Micro Pathology	Biopsy shows **diffuse glomerulonephritis** resulting from proliferation of endothelial, mesangial, and epithelial cells; granular, **"starry-sky" pattern** of IgG, IgM, and C3 on immunofluorescence; electron microscopy shows **subepithelial "humplike" deposits** (antigen-antibody complexes).
Treatment	Penicillin if still infected with *Streptococcus*; diuretics, salt and water restriction and antihypertensives.
Discussion	Poststreptococcal glomerulonephritis is a classic immune complex-mediated entity that is associated with acute nephritic syndrome, which develops following infection with nephritogenic group A β-hemolytic streptococci (e.g., types 1, 4, and 12, which are associated with pharyngitis, and types 49, 55, and 57, which are associated with impetigo).

POSTSTREPTOCOCCAL GLOMERULONEPHRITIS

ID/CC	A **25-year-old male** presents with complaints of sudden-onset **fever** and chills, urgency and burning on micturition (DYSURIA), and perineal pain.
HPI	His symptoms developed a day after he underwent **urethral dilatation** for a stricture.
PE	VS: fever. PE: suprapubic tenderness; rectal exam reveals asymmetrically **swollen**, firm, markedly **tender, hot prostate**; prostatic massage is avoided owing to risk of inducing bacteremia; epididymitis and extreme pain.
Labs	Examination and culture of urine and prostatic secretions reveal ·infection with *Escherichia coli*.
Gross Pathology	Edematous gland enlargement with suppuration of entire gland, possibly abscesses and focal areas of necrosis that have coalesced.
Micro Pathology	Initially minimal leukocytic infiltration of stroma. Later, necrosis of the gland may lead to gland fibrosis.
Treatment	Antibiotic therapy as directed by urine and blood culture sensitivity tests.
Discussion	*Escherichia coli* **is the most common cause** of acute prostatitis; many cases **follow** the use of **instrumentation for the urethra** and prostate (e.g., catheterization, cystoscopy, urethral dilatation, transurethral resection). Remaining infections are caused by *Klebsiella, Proteus, Pseudomonas,* and *Serratia.* Among the gram positives, enterococcus and *Staphylococcus aureus* are frequent causative organisms.

ID/CC	A **65-year-old male** complains of **recurrent burning**, urgency, and **frequency of micturition** together with vague lower abdominal, lumbar, and perineal pain.
HPI	He also complains of a mucoid urethral discharge. He was previously diagnosed via ultrasound with **benign prostatic hypertrophy** but does not report any severe symptoms of prostatism; his medical history reveals **frequent UTIs** due to *Escherichia coli*.
PE	VS: stable; no fever. PE: rectal exam reveals **enlarged, nodular prostate**; biopsy obtained to rule out carcinoma.
Labs	Examination and culture of expressed prostatic secretions reveal leukocytosis and *E. coli*.
Imaging	IVP/voiding cystourethrogram (to rule out underlying anatomic cause): normal.
Gross Pathology	Enlarged prostate with nodularity and calculi.
Micro Pathology	Chronic inflammation and few PMNs around glands and ducts on biopsy; dilated ducts containing inspissated secretions (CORPORA AMYLACEA).
Treatment	**Antibiotics** (TMP-SMX, carbenicillin, quinolones). High fluid intake and abstinence from alcohol. Recurrences are common.
Discussion	Bacterial prostatitis is usually caused by the same gram-negative bacilli that cause UTIs in females; 80% or more of such infections are caused by *Escherichia coli*. Chronic bacterial prostatitis is **common in elderly males** with prostatic hyperplasia and is a frequent cause of recurrent UTIs in males (most antibiotics poorly penetrate the prostate; hence the bacteria are not totally eradicated and continuously seed the urinary tract).

PROSTATITIS—CHRONIC

ID/CC	A 28-year-old black woman who is in her 27th week of pregnancy complains of **right flank pain, high-grade fever**, malaise, headache, and **dysuria**.
HPI	Thus far her pregnancy has been uneventful.
PE	VS: fever. PE: no peripheral edema; **right costovertebral angle tenderness; acutely painful fist percussion on right lumbar area** (POSITIVE GIORDANO'S SIGN).
Labs	CBC: leukocytosis with neutrophilia. UA: proteinuria; hematuria; abundant WBCs and **WBC casts**; pyocytes on sediment; alkaline pH; **urine culture > 100,000 colonies** of *Escherichia coli*.
Imaging	US, renal: slightly enlarged kidney.
Gross Pathology	Kidney enlarged, edematous, and hyperemic with microabscesses in medulla.
Micro Pathology	Pyocytes in tubules; **light blue neutrophils on supravital stain** (GLITTER CELLS); PMN infiltration of interstitium.
Treatment	Antibiotics according to sensitivity; ampicillin; in nonpregnant patients, fluoroquinolone or ampicillin and an aminoglycoside constitute initial treatment.
Discussion	An acute bacterial kidney infection caused mainly by gram-negative bacteria such as *E. coli, Klebsiella, Proteus, and Enterobacter,* acute pyelonephritis usually results from upward dissemination of lower urinary tract bacteria.
Atlas Links	UCVI PG-M2-086A, PG-M2-086B

ID/CC	A 10-year-old female presents with a **high fever, headache, vomiting**, and impaired consciousness.
HPI	She suffered a generalized **seizure** about 45 minutes ago. She was previously diagnosed with **cyanotic congenital heart disease** (ventricular septal defect with Eisenmenger's syndrome).
PE	VS: fever. PE: altered sensorium; **papilledema**; nuchal rigidity; clubbing; **central cyanosis**; cardiac auscultation suggestive of VSD with severe pulmonary arterial hypertension.
Labs	Blood culture reveals **mixed infection** with *Bacteroides*, microaerophilic streptococci, *Staphylococcus aureus*, and *Klebsiella*; staining and culture of pus aspirated from brain abscess confirm polymicrobial infection.
Imaging	CT (with contrast): multiple ring-enhancing lesions with low attenuation centers (ABSCESS) surrounding cerebral edema and ventricular compression.
Gross Pathology	Cavity filled with thick, liquefied pus surrounded by fibrous capsule of variable thickness; pericapsular zone of gliosis and edema.
Micro Pathology	Central portion contains degenerated PMNs and cellular debris; capsule is composed of collagenous fibrous tissue with blood vessels and mixed inflammatory cells.
Treatment	High-dose, extended parenteral broad-spectrum antibiotic coverage; **CT-directed drainage of pus**.
Discussion	Brain abscesses arise secondary to **hematogenous spread** from another infection (bronchiectasis, endocarditis), from contiguous spread from adjacent infection (chronic otitis media, mastoiditis, sinusitis), or following **direct implantation** from trauma. Patients with congenital heart disease with right-to-left shunt are particularly predisposed because the normal filtering action of the pulmonary vasculature is lost.

NEUROLOGY

BRAIN ABSCESS

ID/CC	A 43-year-old male **Mexican** migrant worker visits his ophthalmologist because of pain and **loss of vision** in his right eye.
HPI	Recently he has also suffered from **severe headaches** and **projectile vomiting**.
PE	**Papilledema** on left funduscopic exam; **free-floating cyst** in vitreous body of right eye; chorioretinitis and disk hemorrhage; multiple nontender subcutaneous nodules.
Labs	CBC: eosinophilia. LP: lymphocytic and eosinophilic pleocytosis in CSF with elevated protein and decreased glucose. Eggs of *Taenia solium* in stool sample.
Imaging	XR, plain: small nodular calcifications. CT/MR, brain: characteristic ring-enhancing **intracranial** cysts or calcifications; can cause obstruction and hydrocephalus.
Gross Pathology	Fluid-filled cysts containing scolex surrounded by fibrous capsule in anterior chamber of eye; intraventricular and parenchymal invasion of brain, subcutaneous tissue, and striated muscle.
Micro Pathology	Inflammatory infiltration of cyst by PMNs; necrotic inflammation with calcification upon death of parasite.
Treatment	Surgical removal of parasite from eye; albendazole, corticosteroids/praziquantel for brain disease.
Discussion	Produced by *Cysticercus cellulosae*, the larval form of the pork tapeworm *Taenia solium*, neurocysticercosis is due to the ingestion of ova and spreads through fecal-oral transmission.

ID/CC	A 30-year-old male presents with a **high fever** and chills, **headache, nausea**, vomiting, and muscle aches.
HPI	Yesterday he had an episode involving abnormal movements of his right hand and face (FOCAL SEIZURE). He also has difficulty comprehending speech and has **olfactory hallucinations**. He has no history of psychiatric illness.
PE	VS: fever; tachycardia; mild tachypnea; BP normal. PE: **confused and disoriented; papilledema**; mild nuchal rigidity; Kernig's sign positive; paraphasic errors in speech; deep tendon reflexes normal and bilaterally symmetric.
Labs	LP: cells 400/µL with **mononuclear pleocytosis**; mildly elevated protein; normal glucose; CSF PCR reveals **herpes simplex virus type 1 (HSV-1)**; serum complement-fixing antibody titer > 1:1000. EEG: **spiked and slow waves localized to temporal lobes**.
Imaging	CT: characteristic changes of **encephalitis** seen over **temporal lobes**.
Gross Pathology	Hemorrhagic, necrotizing encephalitis most severe along inferior and medial regions of temporal lobes and orbitofrontal gyri.
Micro Pathology	Brain biopsy reveals **Cowdry intranuclear viral inclusion bodies** in both neurons and glial cells with perivascular inflammatory infiltrates.
Treatment	Intravenous acyclovir.
Discussion	Herpes simplex virus is the **most common cause of acute sporadic encephalitis** in the United States. In the newborn, HSV-2 is usually the cause; after the neonatal period, most cases result from HSV-1. Neonatal infection (usually HSV-2) occurs after exposure to maternal genital infection at the time of delivery. The precise pathogenesis of HSV-1 encephalitis in the older child or the adult is not clear, but viral spread into the temporal lobe by both olfactory and trigeminal routes has been postulated.
Atlas Link	UCV1 M-M2-089

NEUROLOGY

HERPES SIMPLEX ENCEPHALITIS

ID/CC An 11-year-old girl is brought to the ER with high **fever, chills, severe headache, vomiting**, and obtundation.

HPI Her parents report that she suffered a generalized **seizure** about an hour ago. A few days ago, the family had returned from a summer vacation in **south India**, where the child often **played in irrigated rice farms**. She **did not receive any immunizations** prior to her travel.

PE VS: fever. PE: patient is stuporous; neck stiffness and Kernig's sign positive (due to meningeal irritation); mild papilledema; tremors noted in hands.

Labs LP: CSF reveals pleocytosis with **predominant lymphocytosis, mildly elevated proteins, and normal sugar** (suggestive of aseptic meningitis); IgM enzyme immunoassay performed on acute and convalescent sera and CSF reveals significant titer of antibodies to **Japanese encephalitis** virus.

Imaging CT, head: areas of **low density in the thalamus and basal ganglia**.

Treatment Supportive; experimental intrathecal α-interferon therapy.

Discussion Japanese encephalitis virus is a **flavivirus** that causes **disease in humans, horses and pigs**. It is **widely distributed in Asia** from Japan and Eastern Siberia to Indonesia and westward to India; **epidemics** occur in **summer months** coincident with the abundance of the **mosquito vector *Culex tritaeniorhychnus***. The vector breeds in irrigated rice fields and bites preferentially at sunset and sunrise; **pigs are the amplifying hosts**, whereas man is the incidental "dead-end" host. A **vaccine is available** for routine use for childhood immunization in Japan and in developed countries to protect travelers.

ID/CC	A 30-year-old male **laboratory researcher** presents with a **high fever, neck rigidity**, retro-orbital pain, and severe myalgias of a few days' duration.
HPI	The patient also complains of a **sore throat** and photophobia. His work in the lab involves **close contact with** experimental animals such as **hamsters, white mice, and nude mice**. He was adequately vaccinated.
PE	VS: fever. PE: neck stiffness and **Kernig's sign positive** (due to meningeal irritation); pharyngeal inflammation but no exudate noted.
Labs	CBC: mild leukopenia. LP: CSF suggestive of **aseptic meningitis; LCM virus isolated** from CSF. IgG and IgM antibodies detected in serum by immunofluorescent assay.
Treatment	Supportive; ribavirin may play a role.
Discussion	Lymphocytic choriomeningitis virus is an **arenavirus**. Sporadic cases occur after **infection with feral mice**, but the **most common sources** of human infection are **pet/lab rodents**. The virus is considered a **major lab hazard**, and care must be taken to avoid accidental infection. There is **no** commercially available **vaccine**.

LYMPHOCYTIC CHORIOMENINGITIS (LCM)

ID/CC	A 50-year-old white male develops **sudden fever with chills**, pain in the back and extremities, and **neck stiffness**; he vomited six times and had a **convulsion** prior to admission.
HPI	The patient is a **heavy smoker** and is **diabetic. Two weeks ago**, he had a **URI**. He is also very sensitive to light (PHOTOPHOBIA).
PE	Markedly reduced mental status (OBTUNDED); petechial rash over trunk and abdomen; **nuchal and spinal rigidity; positive Kernig's and Brudzinski's signs**; no focal neurologic deficits.
Labs	LP: **elevated pressure; cloudy CSF; elevated protein; markedly decreased glucose; high cell count with mostly WBCs**. CSF Gram stain reveals **gram-positive diplococci**. Spinal fluid culture grows **Streptococcus pneumoniae.**
Imaging	CT/MR, brain: **meningeal thickening** and enhancement.
Gross Pathology	Pia-arachnoid congestion results from inflammatory infiltrate; thin layer of pus forms and promotes adhesions while obstructing normal CSF flow (can cause hydrocephalus); brain covered with purulent exudate, most heavily on base.
Treatment	Early empiric high-dose IV antibiotics; cefotaxime; vancomycin; high-dose steroids.
Discussion	Bacterial meningitis is a pyogenic infection of the CNS that requires prompt treatment. *Streptococcus pneumoniae* is the most common cause of adult meningitis.
Atlas Links	UCV1 PG-M2-092A, PG-M2-092B, M-M2-092 UCV2 NEU-027

ID/CC	A **4-year-old** female presents with a 1-week history of **fever**, severe **headache, irritability**, and **malaise**; 2 days ago she developed **neck stiffness**, and her parents report **projectile vomiting** over the past 24 hours.
HPI	The child is also very sensitive to light (PHOTOPHOBIA). She is fully immunized and has no history of ear, nose, and throat infection, skin rashes, dog bites, or foreign travel.
PE	VS: fever. PE: irritability; resistance to being touched or moved; minimal papilledema of fundus; no focal neurologic signs; no cranial nerve deficits; positive **Kernig's** and **Brudzinski's** signs.
Labs	CBC: **neutrophilic leukocytosis**. LP: increased pressure; **cloudy CSF; neutrophilic pleocytosis; decreased glucose; increased protein; gram-negative coccobacilli**. Negative ZN and India ink staining; normal serum electrolytes; on chocolate agar, blood culture grew *Haemophilus influenzae*; negative Mantoux.
Imaging	CT/MR, brain: **meningeal thickening** and enhancement.
Gross Pathology	Abundant accumulation of purulent exudate between pia mater and arachnoid; meningeal thickening; cloudy to frankly purulent CSF.
Micro Pathology	Intense neutrophilic infiltrate.
Treatment	IV antibiotics (ampicillin, cefotaxime); consider steroids.
Discussion	A pyogenic infection of the nervous system primarily affecting the meninges, bacterial meningitis is most commonly caused by pneumococcus (*Streptococcus pneumoniae*, associated with sickle cell anemia), meningococcus (*Neisseria meningitidis*, associated with a petechial skin rash), and *H. influenzae* (most commonly in children). It is less commonly caused by enterobacteria, *Streptococcus* species, *Staphylococcus* species (due to dental infection), and anaerobic organisms (due to trauma).
Atlas Link	UCV1 M-M2-093

NEUROLOGY

MENINGITIS—BACTERIAL (PEDIATRIC)

ID/CC	A 33-year-old **HIV-positive** white male is brought into the emergency room by his mother because of a **persistent headache**.
HPI	The patient's mother states that her son has been suffering for a long time from **headaches** and **stiff neck** as well as from fever and chills.
PE	VS: fever (39°C). PE: **severe nuchal rigidity**; lack of responsiveness to any command; positive **Kernig's** and **Brudzinski's** signs; diminished patellar and Achilles reflexes; clear lung sounds.
Labs	LP: increased CSF pressure; variable pleocytosis (75 lymphocytes/mm^3); elevated protein; decreased glucose. **Heavily encapsulated, nondimorphic spherical fungal cells** (*CRYPTOCOCCUS NEOFORMANS*) **revealed on India ink staining**; polysaccharide capsular antigen detected on latex agglutination test; diagnosis confirmed by culture on Sabouraud's medium.
Imaging	CT/MR, brain: **multiple ring-enhancing lesions**.
Gross Pathology	Granuloma and abscess formation, mainly at base of brain; CNS primarily affected; lungs affected less commonly.
Micro Pathology	Abundant fungi in CSF and leptomeninges, with slight mononuclear inflammatory reaction; typical **nodular granulomatous meningitis** with exudate.
Treatment	Amphotericin B and 5-flucytosine; fluconazole.
Discussion	Once called torulosis, cryptococcosis is the most common cause of mycotic meningitis; it is acquired through the inhalation of dried **pigeon droppings** and is usually seen in **immunocompromised patients**.
Atlas Link	⬛CⓋ⬛ M-M2-094

MENINGITIS—CRYPTOCOCCAL

ID/CC	A **6-year-old male** being treated for **primary pulmonary tuberculosis** presents with **diplopia**, increasing drowsiness, irritability, and unexplained, recurrent **vomiting**.
HPI	The child has had a low-grade fever, loss of appetite, and a persistent headache over the past few weeks.
PE	VS: fever. PE: stuporous; signs of meningeal irritation noted (**neck rigidity, Kernig's sign**); **CN III and IV palsy** on right side; funduscopy reveals **papilledema**.
Labs	LP (guarded): CSF under **increased pressure** and **turbid**; on standing, a **"cobweb" coagulum** formed at center of tube; CSF studies reveal **lymphocytic pleocytosis**, greatly **elevated protein**, and **low sugar**; ZN staining of CSF coagulum reveals presence of **acid-fast bacilli**; radiometric culture yields *Mycobacterium tuberculosis*.
Imaging	CT: suggests **basal exudates, inflammatory granulomas**, and a **communicating hydrocephalus**; striking meningeal enhancement noted in post-contrast studies.
Gross Pathology	Meningeal surface covered with yellowish-gray exudates and tubercles that are most numerous at base of brain and along the course of the middle cerebral artery; subarachnoid space and arachnoid villi obliterated (leading to poor absorption of CSF and hence a communicating hydrocephalus).
Micro Pathology	Subarachnoid space contains gelatinous exudate of chronic inflammatory cells, obliterating cisterns, and encasing cranial nerves; well-formed **granulomas** occasionally seen, most often at base of brain; arteries running through subarachnoid space show "obliterative endarteritis."
Treatment	Antituberculous therapy with rifampin, isoniazid, ethambutol and pyrazinamide; steroids; ventriculoperitoneal shunt to relieve hydrocephalus.
Discussion	Tuberculous infection reaches the meninges through the hematogenous route, resulting in a clinically subacute form of meningitis; it is often complicated by cranial nerve palsies, a communicating hydrocephalus, decerebrate posturing, convulsions, coma, and death.

NEUROLOGY

ID/CC A 3-year-old male, the child of recent African immigrants, is brought to the local health center because of **asymmetrical legs**.

HPI His parents give a history of **incomplete immunization**. They add that 5 months ago the boy had **fever and diarrhea** that subsided spontaneously; a few weeks later they noted that he could not use his right leg.

PE Right leg **thin, short, wasted, weak, and flaccid; absent deep tendon reflexes** in right leg; **no sensory deficit**; upper limbs normal; mental status and cranial nerves normal.

Labs EMG: chronic partial denervation with abnormal spontaneous activity in resting muscle and reduction in number of motor units under voluntary control; normal sensory conduction studies.

Treatment Rehabilitation, supportive.

Discussion A symptomatic disease caused by poliovirus that is more common in infants and children, poliomyelitis can result in muscular atrophy and skeletal deformity. It attacks motor neurons in the anterior horns and may affect cranial nerves (bulbar polio); it is preventable by vaccine.

ID/CC	A 26-year-old nurse presented with headaches and **recent-onset seizures**; she also complained of increasing **right-sided numbness and blurring of vision**.
HPI	A clinical diagnosis of HSV encephalitis had previously been made, for which the patient was treated with two courses of acyclovir without any amelioration of symptoms; the **disease continued to progress** both radiologically and clinically. On serology she tested **HIV positive**.
PE	Neurologic exam reveals **cognitive mental impairment; visual field defects and sensory dysphasia** seen; **an ill-defined sensory loss** on right side of body.
Labs	HIV positive by ELISA and Western blot.
Imaging	MR (T2-weighted): patchy high-intensity lesions **in the deep white matter of left cerebral hemisphere** involving temporal, parietal, and occipital lobes.
Micro Pathology	Stereotactic biopsy sections show abnormal brain with rarefaction, numerous reactive astrocytes; foamy histiocytes, and inflammatory infiltrate around some vessels; **JC virus in situ hybridization** shows many **positive nuclei**; no herpesvirus inclusions seen; **electron microscopy** demonstrates cells with **typical papovavirus** structures in nucleus.
Treatment	Disease was **relentlessly progressive** and resulted in **death within 6 months**.
Discussion	Progressive multifocal leukoencephalopathy is a **progressive demyelinating disease related to JC papovavirus infection**; the largest number of cases occur in **persons who are immunocompromised** for any of a variety of reasons, including organ transplantation, hematologic and other malignant diseases, chronic immunosuppressive therapy, and AIDS.

PROGRESSIVE MULTIFOCAL LEUKOENCEPHALOPATHY

ID/CC	A 30-year-old male is seen with complaints of a **rash** along with **pain in his left ear** and inability to move the muscles of his face with accompanying asymmetry.
HPI	He suffered an attack of **chickenpox during childhood** but has no history either of a similar rash over his face or of any visual symptoms (to rule out herpes zoster ophthalmicus).
PE	**Vesicular rash** over left pinna (OTITIS EXTERNA); left-sided lower motor neuron-type **facial nerve palsy** (patient is unable to frown and unable to blink left eye; eyeballs roll up during attempt to close eye; patient is unable to whistle; taste sensation over anterior two-thirds of tongue lost on left side).
Labs	Although the diagnosis is predominantly clinical, a **Tzanck test** examining lesion scrapings (showing evidence of multinucleate acantholytic cells), direct culture, and immunohistochemical identification of infected cells allow identification of the virus.
Gross Pathology	Neuritis and vesicular skin lesions confined to distribution of geniculate ganglion of facial nerve.
Micro Pathology	Vesicular skin lesions with **herpes viral inclusions**, i.e., intranuclear, acidophil inclusions with a halo around them (COWDRY TYPE A INCLUSIONS); syncytial cells also seen.
Treatment	**Systemic steroids** are mainstay of management.
Discussion	**Herpes zoster** of the **geniculate ganglion**, or Ramsay Hunt syndrome, presents as a vesicular rash on the pinna followed by ipsilateral LMN facial nerve palsy.

ID/CC	A 30-year-old male presents with a **high fever, neck stiffness**, and **drowsiness**.
HPI	He also complains of nausea and vomiting. He **recently traveled** along the **Mississippi-Ohio River basin**.
PE	VS: fever. PE: **neck stiffness** and **Kernig's sign positive** (due to meningeal irritation); right oculomotor nerve palsy noted; mild papilledema.
Labs	IgM enzyme immunoassay done on paired sera, and CSF confirms the diagnosis of **St. Louis virus** infection. LP: CSF exam reveals pleocytosis with predominant lymphocytosis suggestive of **aseptic meningitis**.
Micro Pathology	Inflammation and neuronal degeneration, principally in the thalamus, midbrain, and brainstem.
Treatment	Supportive treatment.
Discussion	St. Louis encephalitis virus is the **most common cause of epidemic encephalitis** in the United States; cases occur annually as isolated events or in summer and autumn encephalitis epidemics. **Most** infections **are asymptomatic**. The disease occurs throughout the United States, but outbreaks have also occurred in the Caribbean as well as in Central and South America.

ST. LOUIS ENCEPHALITIS

ID/CC   The case of a **12-year-old boy** who **died of a progressive degener-ative neurologic disease** was discussed at an autopsy meeting.

HPI   The child had been developing normally up to 10 years of age, when his teachers noted a **progressive deterioration in intellect and personality**; this was followed by the development of **seizures akin to myoclonus**, signs of pyramidal and extrapyrami-dal disease, and finally a **state of decerebrate rigidity**. The child **died 7 months after the onset** of symptoms. His history revealed that he had had a **severe attack of measles at the age of 2**.

Labs   LP: routine CSF profile normal. **Gamma globulin level elevated**; markedly **elevated levels of measles antibody** present in both serum and CSF; despite the elevated antibody titers, **antibody to the M protein was not present**. EEG: pattern of **burst suppression and biphasic sharp and slow waves**.

Imaging   MR: nonspecific parenchymal abnormalities.

Micro Pathology   Histopathologically, the encephalitis involved both white and gray matter and was marked by lymphocytic infiltration, nerve cell degeneration, and demyelination; measles antigen demon-strated by immunofluorescence analysis, and particles resem-bling paramyxovirus were detected by electron microscopy.

Treatment   No specific therapy available.

Discussion   Subacute sclerosing panencephalitis (SSPE) is caused by a **defective** (major defect is the lack or altered expression of the M-matrix protein) form of **measles virus** (family Paramyxoviridae); SSPE is a **late complication of a measles** infection that is not eliminated from the host. Immunization against measles is the only effective preventive tool.

ID/CC	A 25-year-old **recently married woman** is concerned about a scanty, offensively **malodorous vaginal discharge**.
HPI	She states that the discharge is **thin, grayish-white, and foul-smelling**. She does not complain of vulvar pruritus or soreness.
PE	Pelvic exam confirms presence of a homogenous, grayish-white, watery discharge adherent to the vaginal walls that yields a **"fishy" odor when mixed with KOH**; no injection and excoriation of the vulva, vagina, or cervix.
Labs	Vaginal pH > 5; saline smear reveals presence of **characteristic "clue cells"** (squamous epithelial cells with smudged borders due to adherent bacteria).
Treatment	Single dose of **metronidazole** (2 g) effective in treating the infection. Oral clindamycin is an alternative drug.
Discussion	Although bacterial vaginitis was originally thought to be caused by *Gardnerella vaginalis*, this organism is now recognized to be part of the normal vaginal flora. Bacterial vaginosis is now known to result from a **synergistic interaction of bacteria** in which the normal *Lactobacillus* species in the vagina is ultimately replaced by **high concentrations of anaerobic bacteria**, including ***Bacteroides, Peptostreptococcus, Peptococcus***, and ***Mobiluncus* species** along with a markedly greater number of *G. vaginalis* organisms than is encountered in normal vaginal secretions. Bacterial vaginosis is known to increase the risk of pelvic inflammatory disease, chorioamnionitis, and premature birth.
Atlas Link	UCV1 M-M2-101

ID/CC A 25-year-old puerpera who was **lactating** her week-old infant presents with **pain and swelling** in her left breast.

HPI The symptoms commenced acutely, and she does not recall any previous breast lumps or swellings.

PE **Skin overlying** left breast is **red, edematous, tender, and hot**; area of tense induration felt underlying inflamed skin.

Labs Culture of pus drained from **breast abscess** and **nasopharyngeal swab** taken from the infant grew *Staphylococcus aureus*.

Imaging USG: nearly anechoic area with posterior enhancement.

Treatment **Penicillinase-resistant antibiotic; incision** (in a radial direction over the affected segment) **and dependent drainage** of intra-mammary abscess; breast feeding was temporarily discontinued.

Discussion Bacterial mastitis most commonly occurs in lactating women due to infection of a hematoma or secondary infection of plasma cell mastitis; the infecting **organism is mostly penicillin-resistant *Staphylococcus aureus*.**

ID/CC	A 38-year-old white female visits her gynecologist for a **routine Pap smear**.
HPI	She admits to early sexual activity, **many sexual partners**, and **unprotected sex**.
PE	Pallor; cervical tenderness; a few small, raised, flat lesions on cervix; **genital warts** also seen on vulva (CONDYLOMATA ACUMINATA).
Labs	Presence of HPV in cervical cells revealed on **DNA hybridization and immunofluorescent antibody assays** for viral antigen.
Micro Pathology	Rounded basophilic cells on Pap smear with **large nuclei** occupying most of surface; **nuclei show mitoses and coarse clumping of chromatin with perinuclear halo** (SEVERE KOILOCYTIC DYSPLASIA).
Treatment	Cryotherapy, conization, or local excision with follow-up.
Discussion	Infection with **HPV types 16, 18, and 31** is strongly associated with **cervical cancer** preceded by dysplasia. Spread of the infection to partners may be prevented by barrier contraception.
Atlas Links	UCV1 M-M2-103 UCV2 OB-011A, OB-011B

ID/CC	A 28-year-old **sexually active woman** presents with crampy **lower abdominal pain**, yellowish **vaginal discharge**, and general malaise.
HPI	She also complains of continuous low-grade fever and reveals that the **pain** is **exacerbated during and immediately after menstruation** (CONGESTIVE DYSMENORRHEA). She uses a copper **intrauterine device** for contraception.
PE	VS: low-grade fever. PE: **lower abdominal tenderness**; bimanual pelvic exam demonstrates **purulent vaginal discharge**, bilateral **adnexal tenderness**, and pain on movement of cervix (MUCOPURULENT CERVICITIS).
Labs	CBC: leukocytosis with left shift. Increased ESR; endocervical swab sent for microscopic exam; staining and culture revealed combined infection with *Neisseria gonorrhoeae* (cultured on Thayer-Martin medium) and *Chlamydia trachomatis* (identified on cell culture, immunofluorescence, and antigen capture assay); **laparoscopy** ("gold standard" for diagnosis) confirmed diagnosis.
Imaging	USG: free pelvic fluid, dilated tubular structure in adnexa.
Gross Pathology	Erythema and swelling of fallopian tubes on laparoscopy; seropurulent exudate noted on surface of tubes from fimbriated end.
Micro Pathology	Endocervical swab reveals increased neutrophils and gram-negative diplococci seen both intra- and extracellularly; cervical biopsy reveals inclusions containing *Chlamydia* within columnar cells.
Treatment	Antibiotic therapy with cefoxitin (for *N. gonorrhoeae*) and doxycycline (for chlamydial infection); male partners must be treated for STDs.
Discussion	Pelvic inflammatory disease usually occurs as a primary infection that ascends from the lower genital tract due to STDs caused by *Neisseria gonorrhoeae* and *Chlamydia trachomatis*. Sequelae of PID include peritonitis; intestinal obstruction due to adhesions; dissemination leading to arthritis, meningitis, and endocarditis; chronic pelvic pain; infertility; ectopic pregnancy; and recurrent PID.

ID/CC	A **20-year-old Asian woman** presents with complaints of **infertility** and **heavy bleeding during menses** (MENORRHAGIA).
HPI	She was treated for **pulmonary tuberculosis** a few years ago. She has been unable to conceive despite unprotected intercourse for the past 2 years. Her husband's semen analysis is normal.
PE	On pelvic exam, small, fixed **adnexal masses** are palpable that are matted and fixed to uterus ("FROZEN PELVIS").
Labs	Culture of endometrial curettings yields *Mycobacterium tuberculosis*; histologic examination of curettings reveals presence of **characteristic tubercles**; Mantoux skin test strongly positive.
Imaging	CXR: left apical fibrosis (evidence of old healed pulmonary tuberculosis). (Hysterosalpingography [HSG] is contraindicated in a proven case of tuberculosis. When done in asymptomatic cases, HSG yields certain typical findings, including a **rigid, nonperistaltic, pipelike tube**; beading and variation in filling density; **calcification** of the tube; **cornual block; jagged fluffiness of the tubal outline**; and vascular or lymphatic extravasation of the dye.)
Gross Pathology	Tubes are enlarged, thickened, and tortuous; examination of uterus reveals evidence of **synechiae and adhesions** (leading to **Asherman's syndrome**).
Micro Pathology	Microscopic exam of tubes, ovaries, and endometrium reveals evidence of **granulomas** with giant cells and **caseation**.
Treatment	Four-drug therapy with isoniazid, pyrazinamide, ethambutol, and rifampicin; pyridoxine to prevent isoniazid-induced deficiency.
Discussion	Genital tuberculosis is almost always secondary to a focus elsewhere in the body, with the bloodstream by far the most common method of spread. The fallopian tubes are the most frequently involved part of the genital tract, followed by the uterus. Ninety percent of patients are cured with chemotherapy, although only 10% regain fertility.

PELVIC TUBERCULOSIS

ID/CC A 30-year-old **woman** presents to the ER with an abrupt-onset **high fever, vomiting, profuse diarrhea**, severe muscle aches, and disorientation.

HPI One day ago she developed an **extensive skin rash** all over her body. Her husband says she used a **vaginal sponge** for contraception.

PE VS: fever; tachycardia; hypotension. PE: extremely toxic-looking; drowsy but responding to verbal commands; **extensive scarlatiniform rash** seen involving entire body; pharyngeal, conjunctival, and vaginal mucosa congested (frank hyperemia); no neck rigidity or Kernig's sign demonstrable; funduscopic exam normal; no localizing neurologic deficits.

Labs CBC: leukocytosis; thrombocytopenia. UA: mild pyuria (in absence of UTI). BUN and creatinine elevated; blood cultures sterile; **culture of cervical secretions grows *Staphylococcus aureus*.** LP: CSF normal. Serology for Rocky Mountain spotted fever, leptospirosis, and measles negative.

Treatment **Vigorous IV fluids** and parenteral **penicillinase-resistant penicillin** or first-generation cephalosporins; patient in this case recovered, and typical skin desquamation was seen over palms and soles during convalescence.

Discussion Toxic shock syndrome results from infection with *Staphylococcus aureus*. Its effects are mediated through the **exotoxin TSST-1**, which functions as a superantigen, stimulating the production of interleukin-1 and tumor necrosis factor. Staphylococcal TSS has been associated with the use of **vaginal contraceptive sponges** and with many types of localized staphylococcal soft tissue infections. Most cases of TSS occur in **menstruating women**.

Atlas Links ⬜🅄🄲🅅2 OB-027A, OB-027B

ID/CC A 28-year-old primigravida at 36 weeks' gestation presents with a **high fever**.

HPI She was being monitored following a **premature rupture of the membranes**.

PE VS: **fever**; fetal tachycardia. PE: **uterine tenderness**.

Labs Elevated maternal total lymphocyte count; **vaginal swab** culture revealed colonization with **group B streptococcus**.

Treatment Presence of group B streptococcus in vagina after premature rupture of membranes was an indication for **immediate delivery and treatment of the infant**; mother was also treated with **intravenous antibiotics**.

Discussion A significant proportion of the population is colonized in the vagina and rectum with **group B streptococcus, which is correlated with preterm labor, premature rupture of membranes** (PROM), **chorioamnionitis, and neonatal sepsis**; neonates with group B streptococcus sepsis have a 25% mortality rate. Among preterm neonates, this figure doubles to over 50%; therefore **antibiotic prophylaxis** is recommended in the setting of **preterm delivery and PROM** even without the diagnosis of frank chorioamnionitis. When chorioamnionitis is suspected, intravenous antibiotics are started and delivery is hastened.

ID/CC	An 8-month-old male infant is brought to a pediatrician because of severe, intractable **chronic diarrhea** and **failure to thrive**.
HPI	The **mother died of AIDS** shortly after the baby was delivered. The baby was **asymptomatic at birth**.
PE	VS: fever; tachycardia. PE: emaciated, grossly malnourished; **oral thrush; generalized lymphadenopathy; hepatosplenomegaly**.
Labs	**Decreased CD4+ cell count**; increased serum immunoglobulin level with impaired production of specific antibodies; **ELISA and Western blot for HIV-1 positive** (could be due to placental transfer of antibodies to HIV, but strongly supports diagnosis in presence of symptoms); PCR for **HIV RNA positive** (confirming HIV infection).
Treatment	Nutritional support, *Pneumocystis carinii* prophylaxis, azidothymidine (ZIDOVUDINE, or AZT) therapy (suppresses replication by inhibiting viral reverse transcriptase), and anti-infective agents for specific infections; IV serum immunoglobulin to reduce frequency of bacterial infections; **oral polio vaccine and BCG contraindicated**.
Discussion	Vertical transmission of HIV-1 may occur in utero through **transplacental passage** of the virus, **during delivery**, or **postnatally through breast feeding**; however, it is believed that most infections are acquired at birth through contact with contaminated blood or secretions. Women who carry the virus should thus be discouraged from becoming pregnant or from breast feeding. The rate of transmission of HIV-1 from mother to infant has varied from 13% to 45%, with an average of 25%; however, when AZT is administered to HIV-1-infected pregnant women and to infants during the first 6 weeks of life, the risk of maternal-infant transmission is significantly reduced.

ID/CC	A 4-year-old white male presents with fever, chills, malaise, **pain**, and **immobility of the right knee** of 1 week's duration.
HPI	Two weeks ago the child fell while playing, but no abnormality was found by the school nurse.
PE	Overlying skin **warm and red; swelling** of distal third of thigh and knee; **tenderness** on palpation.
Labs	CBC: leukocytosis. **Elevated ESR**. Gram stain and culture confirm diagnosis and isolate pathogen.
Imaging	XR, plain: early findings include soft tissue edema and thin line running parallel to diaphysis **(periosteal thickening)**; later findings include bone erosion, subperiosteal abscess with periostitis, and sequestrum formation (due to detached necrotic cortical bone); involucrum formation (laminated periosteal reaction). MR: marrow edema; abscess. Indium-labeled WBC, scan: hot spot.
Gross Pathology	**New osteoblastic periosteal bone formation** (INVOLUCRUM); **trapping of detached necrotic bone by involucrum** (SEQUESTRUM); isolated localized abscess (BRODIE'S ABSCESS); sinus tract formation, draining pus to skin.
Micro Pathology	Purulent exudate formation, usually metaphyseal, with ischemic necrosis of bone due to increased pressure of pus in rigid bone walls; vascular thrombosis.
Treatment	IV antibiotics according to sensitivity; **surgical debridement**.
Discussion	Osteomyelitis is an acute pyogenic bone infection which, if left untreated, produces functional incapacity and deformities. The most common pathogen is *Staphylococcus aureus*; less frequently *Streptococcus* and enterobacteria are involved. In sickle cell anemia *Escherichia coli* and *Salmonella* species are seen; diabetics are at risk for *Pseudomonas* infection. Immunocompromised patients may show *Sporothrix schenckii* osteomyelitis; human bites, anaerobes; puncture wounds, *Pseudomonas aeruginosa*; and cat-bite wounds, *Pasteurella multocida*.

ID/CC	A 21-year-old female college student complains of low-grade fever along with **pain** and **swelling** in the left knee of 5 days' duration.
HPI	She had been to her family physician 2 weeks ago because of **dysuria** and a **purulent vaginal discharge** (due to gonococcal infection) and was given an "antibiotic shot". She was asymptomatic until 4 days ago. She then developed **fever, chills**, and pain in both wrists and in her left ankle, which disappeared when the pain appeared in her left knee (MIGRATORY POLY-ARTHRALGIA).
PE	Swollen, tender, warm left knee with **limited range of motion**; white vaginal discharge.
Labs	Intracellular, bean-shaped gram-negative diplococci (GONOCOCCI) and **markedly elevated WBC count** on urethral smear and **synovial fluid aspirate** culture of synovial aspirate grows gonococci.
Imaging	XR, knee: soft tissue swelling.
Treatment	IV ceftriaxone.
Discussion	Almost always accompanied by synovitis and effusion, gonococcal arthritis can rapidly destroy articular cartilage and is often associated with skin rash and C5, C6, C7, and C8 complement deficiencies. Single joints are usually affected, most often the wrists, fingers, knees, and ankles.